MEDICAL MADNESS

MEET THE GOLDEN RULE

GEORGE HUBER

authorHOUSE®

AuthorHouse™ LLC
1663 Liberty Drive
Bloomington, IN 47403
www.authorhouse.com
Phone: 1-800-839-8640

Published by AuthorHouse 09/29/2014

ISBN: 978-1-4969-1979-3 (sc)
ISBN: 978-1-4969-1980-9 (hc)
ISBN: 978-1-4969-1978-6 (e)

Library of Congress Control Number: 2014916473

Contents

Foreword

About the Author

The delicate yet invasive nature of this subject makes it very important for you, the reader, to know me—without my exposing those whose privacy is essential due to ethical, moral, and legal considerations.

A tiny town with great people, located along the beautiful but temperamental and at times rampaging, Ohio River, New Richmond, population under 2,600, just twenty miles east of Cincinnati, was my birthplace and home through my childhood until my late teens. I was very close, in my youth, to an African American friend living less than a block away. We often walked to and from school together. I cherished that relationship inasmuch as it helped to inoculate me from the deep prejudice prevalent in much of the country. I looked up to him and still do. He was quite good at most anything he attempted—and outstanding in whatever he committed himself to. He became highly regarded as a singer, to the extent that he was often invited to sing the National Anthem for the Cincinnati Reds, the dominant major league baseball team in the area. We remain close to this day.

My father died tragically of a heart attack just a week prior to my high school graduation. The shock had a numbing effect on me; I coped by going through the motions, pretending to be involved.

Curiously, as now I recall, our superintendent was away due to an emergency, and our diplomas could not be signed, so our class of twenty-five received a blank sheet of paper until the official diplomas were prepared. As we ascended the stage for that ceremony, three rows of chairs were arranged, just two chairs short of the number of graduating students. Those of us in the back row took turns kneeling down, pretending to be seated, as speakers heralded our optimistic future. One student began a humorous chant, low enough to be heard only by those in our little class: "No diplomas. No chairs." The giggling was contagious.

During those years, I met and married my wife, my childhood sweetheart, who continues to be my most trusted friend and partner in everything we do. Following my public school enrollment in elementary and high school, I moved to Cincinnati, where a great deal of my early college work was completed. During this period, my wife and I were blessed with three wonderful children, a daughter and two sons, who have enriched our lives beyond anything we could ever have dreamed.

In 1954, I enrolled in the Cincinnati Christian University (then the Cincinnati Bible Seminary) where I explored in further depth my emergent interest in religion. In 1958, I was awarded an AB degree, followed by a ThB (bachelor of theology degree) in 1959. I enrolled in the University of Cincinnati in 1963 and was awarded an M.Ed in 1966. Later that year, I entered the University of Florida, where I majored in counseling and psychology. I was awarded an EdS degree in 1970. I continued to pursue advanced graduate work at the University of Florida (UF) while enjoying an extended tenure at Santa Fe College.

My immersion in the college atmosphere was exciting. Santa Fe was a very young, vibrant institution, founded as a community college in 1966. I was very fortunate to be hired as a full-time instructor in the fall of 1968. My role was first as an instructor in the behavioral sciences, followed by my assignment as director of counseling. I had the privilege of supervising more than a dozen internship students from the University of Florida, at times two or three per term, who were pursuing graduate study and doctoral programs. They were also my teachers via that intense, shared learning environment.

The challenge of the university curriculum, along with my engagement in a new, animated college, which became nationally known for its innovative programs, left little time for outside interests. In addition to my own teaching and studies, I was elected President of the Faculty Association at Santa Fe in 1969. It was a challenging and stirring period, given the social and political upheaval in America, whose barometer of turbulence was located on college campuses. That period was referred to succinctly as "the sixties."

You may determine from the title of this book and its focus up to this point that the emphasis on the Golden Rule flows naturally from a theological perspective, and that may well be the case for those who so choose. But it will be less so in this context because the maxim derives from many cultures, and I do not wish it to be limited to a narrow sectarian context—its sources are multiple and universally inclusive.

My Mentors

If you come upon a turtle atop a fence post, you know immediately that it did not get there by itself—a touch of modern political humor from a variety of sources. Seriously, I take full responsibility for my own shortcomings. A key aspect of success is sharing credit with the creators of inspiration and counsel from which one has benefited immensely.

My exceptional strength in educational pursuits came from two crucial encounters with the most talented men I have ever met. Good fortune smiled on me early in having these two remarkably gifted and generous mentors during my educational, religious, and social endeavors in academic communities. They complemented each other in their diverse contributions and influence on me, and provided an incredible balance of conservative and progressive influences on my development; that balance is reflected in this presentation of my subsequent challenging medical experience, which prompted this book.

Mentor Number One

Dr. Lewis Foster (BD, Yale Divinity School; STM, Harvard Divinity School; PhD in history and philosophy of religion, Harvard School of Arts and Sciences) was a professor and mentor whose instruction I treasure. I was privileged to enroll in his classes while pursuing my ThB, and thereafter I frequently sought his counsel in founding a campus student ministry for members of our denomination as they pursued their studies at Miami University of Ohio. Dr. Foster can be reasonably referred to as a religious conservative or fundamentalist, who was respected and admired even by those who embraced a different religious focus and philosophy. He had a firm commitment to intellectual honesty and was willing to explore that map of scholarship wherever it led. He knew who he was, what he believed, and why, and he was most generous with his time and intellectual engagement. I recall an interesting and revealing incident that discloses the dynamism of academic communities affecting students' lives.

As president of the local ministerial association (a yearly appointment), I announced at one of our regular monthly meetings that we were inviting Dr. Foster to speak to our students. The talk would be open to all and tailored to the concerns of both students and faculty. I then said, "He holds graduate degrees from Yale and Harvard and has his PhD from Harvard—and he is a fundamentalist."

One of the very kind local pastors responded without hesitation, "That's impossible!" He intended no criticism or unkindness, but the limitations of his own personal experience left him a bit befuddled. Obviously, his understanding was more limited regarding the varieties of religious scholarship and commitment.

Dr. Foster came as scheduled, and two hundred or so students and faculty attended. It was a great evening for all.

On a few occasions I was invited to speak at my alma mater, Cincinnati Christian University, for their scheduled chapel services, which I really enjoyed. Dr. Foster was one of several extraordinary scholars on the faculty of this small but vibrant Christian University. On one occasion my presentation was entitled, "The Pursuit of Happiness." It was especially well received, and Dr. Foster invited me to draft it into an essay format to be published in the *Seminary Review*.[1] My brief introduction in the preface of this publication outlines my role at Oxford, Ohio: "Mr. Huber is a leader in the University Christian Fellowship of Oxford, Ohio, organized to supply a campus ministry for Miami University and Western College for Women. His interest in the university student is seen in this message delivered in one of the Chapel Services."

My close relationship with Dr. Foster was further reflected in two articles I published in the *Christian Standard*.[2] On my article about the campus ministry, the magazine reported, "Dr. Lewis Foster said, as we were discussing our program with him, 'This is one of the greatest needs of our churches today.'"

This same publication, the *Christian Standard*,[3] was and continues to be a vital publication for the locally autonomous churches relying on it for receiving information and sharing common interests, programs, and projects.

My purpose in listing these articles is to affirm for the reader my level of commitment to engaging the minds of students as they formulated plans for their lives in demanding academic communities.

Mentor Number Two

Dr. Roy Ward, who held a bachelor of sacred theology (STB) degree and a doctor of theology (ThD) degree from Harvard

---

[1] George Huber, "The Pursuit of Happiness," *Seminary Review* X, no. 2 (Winter 1964).

[2] George Huber, "The Church Faces a Never-Again Opportunity and Obligation to Serve on the University Campus," *Christian Standard* 516 (August 18, 1962): 4.

[3] George Huber, "The Need for A Campus Ministry," *Christian Standard* 23 (January 11, 1964): 7–8.

University, was my next mentor. He became professor of comparative religion and later associate provost at Miami University in Oxford, Ohio. His career began in 1964. Dr. Ward, upon hearing of our student religious foundation there, contacted me, and asked if he could join us in this endeavor. He did not have to repeat his request. He and I worked together on this important program until I left to continue my studies at the University of Florida. His influence on us was beyond what any academician could have expected to wield.

He possessed an understanding of the future direction of social diversity and harmony that was prescient, surpassing that of anyone I have ever met. His philosophy, even in those early years, was that of inclusion. He wisely cautioned that, if one decides to exclude, "make sure your decision is not based on your own prejudice." That invited a process of self-examination that I have valued to this day. He was a voice for those whose voices weren't heard. He was an early member of the National Organization for Women in Oxford. He was a life member of the NAACP, and as associate provost he frequently advocated for LGBT faculty and students in this conservative university serving upper-middle-class students.

Here I must share a most remarkable experience: On Sunday, June 3, 2012, at about 1:00 p.m., as my wife and I were finishing lunch, we reminisced about Roy's contribution to our work. The discussion centered on whether Roy had participated with us during a period when some other friends, with quite differing philosophies, had been active with us at that time. I told her I would check with him and see what he remembered.

I finished lunch and went to my computer to contact Roy. The message on his website was his obituary. A memorial service at the beautiful Sesquicentennial Chapel on the campus of Miami

University in Oxford, Ohio, was scheduled for 1:30 p.m. that same afternoon. I am not the most emotionally expressive person; however, on this occasion, the tears flowed down my cheeks. I sat there without speaking for several minutes with a panorama of vivid images moving in sequence around me. Recovering my composure, I hurried an e-mail message expressing my condolences to his family. I was transfixed in memory by the likeness of the beautiful chapel where I had officiated marriage rites for several student couples. I'm not superstitious, nor a confirmed mystic—but I know I was nudged to share in that transitional event.

These two men played a significant role in my life. I mention them because I want to show how their contribution to my work provided me with the incentive, discipline, and research capacity necessary to create this book.

Prologue

It was a beautiful Saturday, made especially for tennis! Mid-November's idyllic weather was tantalizing. The day was a replica of so many others I had shared with my tennis friend. The leaves were green, tan, bronze, and golden; the weather in the South was mild. We both relished playing and enjoyed each other's company. My partner (a hand surgeon) and I (a retired educator) played regularly on Saturdays for several years. Early mornings were ideal since my partner was often on call at a local hospital. Professional interruptions were less frequent in the early hours.

An ominous medical cloud loomed on my horizon. I was apprehensive and could not shake it. I had scheduled surgery for prostate cancer the coming Monday. Diagnosed in midsummer, I had shared the news with no one except my wife and children.

We elected to have a radical prostatectomy with the assistance of the celebrated da Vinci robot, a recently designed innovation. It was to be minimally invasive and was then regarded as a major medical advance. My biopsy, found to be positive, was followed immediately by a second opinion from a premier medical center to verify the diagnosis. I had investigated the procedure as well as the surgeon as thoroughly as possible. Experts were supportive. An internationally recognized traditional surgeon spoke favorably of the procedure, the surgeon, and the hospital's performance. He asserted, "We're among the best in the country."

My Last Tennis Match

Little did I realize that my apprehension was prescient. I write this, nearly five years removed, knowing now that was to be my last tennis match—my last chance to relish robust health. I was a fitness enthusiast, enjoyed planned vacations, and relished the numerous pleasures for which good health is a prime prerequisite. The upcoming procedure was destined to be a life-altering trauma, the unexpected and dramatic termination of life as I had come to know it.

This narrative offers a patient's perspective. As we may well expect, there are numerous articles and books by medical professionals, yet there are very few by patients documenting their own personal experiences. This I will guarantee: your understanding of my experience will drastically change your perception of our medical system. Experiencing the system through me, you may be less certain, less trusting, more perceptively critical, but also safer. You will be introduced to the current medical reality. So read on! The life you save may be your own—or one even more precious to you. This, as I will suggest, could have been you, your father, or your son. What happened to me is happening all over our great country even as I write.

You need all the information you can get. If you ever face medical procedures, my experience may become helpful in guiding you. You will have been there, so to speak, before it happens—and it is coming—always sooner than you think. What you don't know about your upcoming hospital stay can kill you. What I am sharing with you may well help save your life. In the medical arena, ignorance and blind trust are a miscalculation when dealing with a profession so plagued by mistakes—unwitting but deadly—and so effective at well-practiced concealment.

Thinking I'll Be Back—Wasn't to Be

I shared the news of this impending surgery with my tennis friend, since it would put our favorite long-standing hobby on hold. I had reason at the time to anticipate—in fact, expect—that with the minimally invasive procedure I had selected, if all went as planned, it would be Saturday tennis as usual in a few months. That was not to be. This ominous, fleeting interruption proved to be horrendously permanent. I never got to hit another tennis ball after that surgery. As I sit here, above my shoulder, to the right, highly visible, on the top shelf of my closet are four cans of unopened, aging tennis balls, a constant, observable reminder of my disenchanted expectations.

Relating this experience brings a disquieting mixture of catharsis, rumination, and reflection. I decided it's better to write and disclose for the good of all—I have come to regard this sharing as an opportunity and obligation. What I discovered as a patient is now being validated by numerous medical professionals. They have recently begun to flood the literature, which brings a ray of hope. To confirm their commitment to a brighter future, many narratives read like penitent confessions disclosing these professionals' own past complicities, failures, and personal wrongs in the practice, and their previous refusal to reveal openly having witnessed appalling behavior by their colleagues. They have begun to tell the truth about the negative impact of the long, corrosive influence of this concealment.

There is another side to the coin of our medical experience. I have no professional obligation regarding issues in the medical profession, as do medical professionals who may have been party to perpetuating the faulty system, if only by remaining silent in the face of avoidable tragedies and who have thereby become willing partners in this culture of concealment. I have not endorsed that unspoken institutional oath of silence. But as I have said, to the credit of some, this is beginning to change. To the more conscientious among them, it was clearly intolerable to keep silent any longer. My commitment is moral and ethical, motivating me to share the unvarnished truth from my perspective as a patient. I bear no responsibility for the system's reckless commitment to the cult of secrecy, as serious malpractice has been inflicted and shrouded by mutually complicit silence.

Chapter One

Our Medical System, Badly Broken

How bad is it? We will hear just how bad it is from leading professionals serving in some of the most prestigious medical institutions in our country—take a listen!

Dr. Marty Makary rivets our attention with the designation, omerta, qualifying and lamenting his medical experiences in numerous hospitals. It brings images of carnage, unintended but institutionally endorsed. A medical mafia was ready to protect its turf by immoral obedience of loyalty and concealment in any case. Focusing on a representative patient with breast cancer he illustrates how life and death choices are, in this hallowed field, incredibly corrupt--and patients die as a result. There are excellent medical opportunities nearby in this and many such cases--but the code of silence and concealment enforced by the system prevent routinely good people from doing the right thing for patients and sounding cautionary alarms. Medical morality, as seen through his eyes, illuminates for us what lurks in the dark shadows camouflaged by medical mythology. He writes:

> "Not for the first time in my career, I felt the weight of ethics on my shoulders like an incubus. I desperately wanted to tell Gretchen to go elsewhere. But I did not. I knew that referring her elsewhere would violate the resident's code of omerta and get me in big trouble, and maybe even fired....I rotated through more departments....neurosurgery, ear- nose- and throat, and urology (about fifty rotations in all) and five more hospitals...When I try

to forgive myself for failing Gretchen, I think I had good reasons at the time...."

As a surgeon now at Johns Hopkins Medical Center, he relates these episodes in his recent book, *Unaccountable*.[4] Makary offers a searing indictment from the inside, arguing that the modern health-care industry, unlike almost every other, doesn't disclose its performance or pricing practices to the public and keeps under wraps information about mistakes and substandard quality. For instance, he discusses such commonsense procedures as hand hygiene, or the lack thereof.

Given the impact infections have in medical treatment, hand hygiene should have fixed rules and consequential regulations. That we are now, so late in our understanding of bacterial and viral safety precautions, having to force otherwise reputable hospitals to do what should be second nature seems deplorable. That there is a risk of the increased probability of killer infections spreading as a result of the abandonment of medical common sense should be inconceivable. Recently, North Shore University Hospital on Long Island realized that health care professionals perform this essential life-saving ritual as little as 30 percent of the time, and the facility took action to correct this shortcoming.

The federally run Centers for Disease Control and Prevention note that hospital-acquired infections cost $30 billion, with a mortality rate of one hundred thousand people per year. The article, "With Money at Risk,"[5] describes new procedures that have been instituted

---

4   Marty Makary, *Unaccountable: What Hospitals Won't Tell You and How Transparency Can Revolutionize Health Care* (New York: Bloomsbury Press, 2012). Pp. 60-61
5   Anemona Hartcollis, "With Money at Risk, Hospitals Push Staff to Wash Hands, *New York Times*, May 29, 2013.

to ensure patient safety. Some of these include sensors alerting video cameras, hand-washing coaches, and forfeiture of Medicare money. Doctors, despite being authority figures, are sometimes the most serious violators, prompting the use of buttons that say, "Ask me if I've washed my hands," thereby burdening patients' relatives with a responsibility that should be insisted upon by the administration. This is so important to the hospital environment. We will address this issue in greater detail in a later section, "Follow the Money."

Medical Miscues

Brilliant Youth Dead in Three Days

Disregarding these essential procedures recently resulted in the death of an aspiring young man. His life was snuffed out because those entrusted with his care were not doing a sufficiently meticulous job in light of the awesome responsibility assigned them. This innocent young life was cut tragically short by a failure to do something as basic as interpret his blood profile results before his hospital dismissal. A raging infection that could have been arrested resulted in his death within three days. Now the prominent hospital has implemented a checklist (too late for our young man) that will, hopefully, result in their being forced routinely to pay attention.

Maureen Dowd, dramatically relates the tragic consequences of medical errors that resulted in the death of this very bright twelve-year-old boy:

> Every parent's nightmare unfolded at warp speed, as the Web site Everyday Health reported and as Jim Dwyer heartbreakingly revealed in Thursday's Times. Rory might have been saved by a swift dose of antibiotics but instead perished in a perfect storm of

false assumptions, overlooked data and overburdened doctors. . . . [Lab tests showed] abnormal production of white blood cells, a sign that infection could be raging, but that red flag was ignored.

"If something good comes from Rory's death, it will be that we realize we have a broken system," he [Jim Dwyer] told me. "Patient care is so fragmented. . . . Medical professionals aren't taught these human skills. . . . So there's insufficient sharing of information and ineffective communication ... They're inexcusable and unthinkable.[6]

It's too easy to lose tabs on elderly patients as well. They are usually frailer and often possess multiple maladies, any one of which may prove terminal if not given vigilant attention. Their mixture of medications and the requirement to be physically attentive to oversee their needs requires more staff time and heightened sensitivity. Articles and books are appearing more often, authored by relatives of loved ones who have been lost to the system, who slipped through the cracks when they should have recovered and enjoyed many more of their twilight years.

One such close call was reported by an ER physician, who is also a medical editor, describing her own personal experience. Managing a busy schedule and covering a hectic assignment, she described her patient as a nonagenarian (in her nineties) whom she then easily stereotyped as demented. This appeared to be a logical diagnosis, quite fitting given the need to process the woman expeditiously under the hospital's chaotic conditions. Essential tests were carried out, but under the stress of the patient load, important but routine available test data was ignored. The prognosis was made via assumptions based on the patient's age and demeanor. A CT scan, critical to an accurate diagnosis, was not read, and in fact was assumed to be normal.

---

[6]   Maureen Dowd, "The Boy Who Wanted to Fly," *New York Times,* July 14, 2012.

Intracranial bleeding was missed by our too-busy physician, and if it had not been caught by others, the bleeding would most likely have killed this patient. I surmise from the account that this ER, which is a replica of so many, will be a death trap for some unlucky patient who will not have the fortunate backup to prevent the tragic consequences of a hasty mistake. This cries out for organizational scrutiny. Compelling incentives must come from without. I have chosen to let the doctor tell you in her own words what happened and how she felt about it. Please note the role of the persistent habit of practiced concealment, which the medical profession says it is trying desperately to change. She writes:

> I quickly scanned through the labs, called the ward's doctor and ran through the case—demented patient, still demented, return to nursing home tomorrow.
>
> I remember the doctor's voice so clearly: "You're sure the labs and everything are normal?" Yes, yes, I said, everything is fine. She hesitated, then said O.K. The intern and I high-fived each other, and bolted back to our other admissions. [*Note from the book's author: she lied to her superior here.*]
>
> The next afternoon the doctor tracked me down. Without mincing words, she told me that she'd been called overnight by the radiologist; the patient's head CT showed an intracranial bleed. The patient was now with the neurosurgeons, getting the blood drained from inside her skull.
>
> I had failed to check the head CT! I was appalled at myself, mortified by my negligence. I stumbled through the rest of the day, an acrid mix of shame and guilt churning inside me.
>
> I never told anyone about my lapse—not my intern, not my attending physician, certainly not the patient's family. I tried to rationalize it: the radiologist had caught the bleeding, and no additional harm had come to the patient. But the instinct for most medical professionals is to keep these shameful mistakes to ourselves. [7]

---

[7]   Danielle Ofri, "My Near Miss" (op-ed), *New York Times*, May 29, 2013.

The doctor announces via this article to thousands of readers how the plague of concealment is destroying the integrity and effectiveness of the medical profession—burying malpractice is still silent killing. *Shameful* is hardly a strong enough adjective to convey what is routinely a part of this tragic system. She felt she must not tell the patient's family. The institution could not tolerate that level of integrity. Suppose the patient under the care of such distracted medical professionals had been this doctor's mother—I believe she would want to know about this. A Golden Rule ethic would bring us much closer to a level of compassionate behavior we can live with.

Doctors who recognize how easy it is to make mistakes have taken to calling for better care and more specific procedures to prevent simple problems from becoming major mistakes. The *Wall Street Journal* reports, "As medical director for Johns Hopkins University's Center for Innovation in Quality Patient Care, Peter Pronovost, 46, has spent most of his career as a champion of innovative but practical solutions to fix system flaws that can lead to deadly mistakes and complications in hospitals.

"Dr. Pronovost's current crusade is preventing deadly bloodstream infections linked to central lines or catheters used in intensive-care units. . . . He hasn't shied away from criticizing his peers for resisting safety and quality improvement efforts." Pronovost explained in a 2011 interview with author Laura Landro:

> The pilot who neglects a checklist before take-off would not be allowed to fly, and most safe industries have transgressions that are firing offenses. . . . But there hasn't been that kind of accountability in health care.
> Nurses and pharmacists work for the hospital, which typically has clear lines of authority and procedures for

dealing with failure to follow accepted practices. But physicians are often self-employed, have little training in teamwork and, perhaps like all of us, are often overconfident about the quality of care they provide, believing things will go right rather than wrong. Nurses are often reluctant to question them, and hospitals don't pressure physicians about teamwork for fear of jeopardizing the business they bring to the hospital.

He also described his latest attempts to improve medical care by addressing the issue of deadly infections.

A pilot project in Michigan showed that participating hospitals reduced rates of infections and death by using a checklist of evidence-based steps to reduce the infections—and by fostering a culture of safety and teamwork.

Dr. Pronovost's boyish appearance and enthusiastic manner belie a steely determination to challenge the status quo in medicine."[8]

A Patient's Perspective

I'm a serial patient and very lucky to be alive to share this experience and help prevent medical errors from plaguing you. In this book, I recount provocative discussions and comments, both positive and negative, with and from medical professionals. Patients' experiences can assist by providing vital information that will enhance medical progress. Concealment covers errors at an enormous cost in patients' lives and precludes medical advancement by curtailing vital learning that could be gained from the shared analysis of failures. In fairness to patients, accountability is essential, and acknowledging mistakes is a no-brainer for those who wish to

---

[8] Laura Landro, "The Secret to Fighting Infections: Laura Landro Interviews Peter Pronovost," *Wall Street Journal,* March 30, 2011.

progress. Our firsthand experiences recount extraordinary situations, inconceivable rationalizations (excuses), and maneuvers to conceal mistakes.

A routine surgical procedure, performed poorly (my appraisal), with complications (the official assessment), sentenced me to four additional surgeries, three in the first year, with each one more serious, more dangerous, and more debilitating than the preceding one. Each of the ensuing medical encounters made the need for subsequent surgeries more probable, more essential. As I write this I am still recuperating, only a few months past the most recent surgery. This proved to be the most devastating, leaving me with a temporary colostomy, which soon prolapsed dangerously—exposing four to six inches of my colon whenever I was up and about. It retreated only when I reclined flat on my back at night. This complication made further surgery essential. I chose to have what is referred to in medical parlance as a "takedown," to enable me, hopefully, to resume more routine bowel functions.

Defense by Denial

A commitment to transparency challenges defense by denial. I must alert readers that, from my experience, concealment was the unspoken order of the day——and it will soon be clear why. Burying mistakes is a common practice, according to disclosing professionals. Hiding this practice requires a vast system of repression and subjugation at all levels of an organization. A systemic change from the top down, a genuine commitment to transparency at all levels of medical practice, is being called for repeatedly by medical professionals, as you have just read. This commitment should have been in existence long ago. I am recounting what I experienced, and it is shocking but not inconsistent with what the professionals themselves are now openly acknowledging. I no longer fear a challenge to my credibility on these issues.

The Hospital in Your Future

We focus on the system, following the lead confirmed by numerous medical professionals and validated by my personal experience and that of many others, and one that will one day be verified by yours. It is understandable, though not justifiable. The hospital in your future harbors incredible dangers created by an environment that is more fully understood when viewed in the light of its relationships with Wall Street, Main Street, and No Harm Street.

Chapter Two

Wall Street, Main Street, No Harm Street

It may seem a bit of a stretch to conjoin these three pillars of our culture. It is helpful to see how and why patients may be treated as third-class citizens and why the system inside and out must become more patient- centered and bring about necessary receptive changes. From the outset you may find it sobering that transparency is being invoked as an antidote for all three systems. I know from my own experience what may well be in store for you and your family unless our society, the medical community, and we ourselves can remake that system. Medical professionals are now spearheading their own effort and urging incentives be applied to do just that. I trust my medical encounters can be a contributing voice of experience and add to this essential mission. The problem is primarily systemic which becomes clear upon examination.

My hope for you and yours is that you will get the best care possible when you become a patient. Unfortunately, now, from what the professionals tell us, being a medical patient does not come with a guarantee of trust and assurance, and that expectation should be moderated. We will all get sick and need that vital help. It can and should be markedly safer and better than it is now.

My book is an attempt to help facilitate better medical outcomes for all of us. This narrative is informative. It is true, since I have nothing to hide; therefore, it may be frightening, depressing, astonishing, and at times humorous, and will be vital for those who choose to learn from another patient's medical voyage.

The most encouraging development is that the books and articles challenging the medical establishment are from the pens of medical professionals, primarily physicians and surgeons. Their tone has shifted to a willingness to share in that drastic change of direction openly. Their increasing numbers are quite critical. They are saying uniformly, *Our hospitals must stop killing people!* I applaud their newly embraced openness, and as a patient I'm contributing a viewpoint that validates their position.

While their strategy is evolving their mission is not fully accomplished, the need is obvious. Agreement resides in this premise: our medical system faces serious systemic deficiencies. Common folks need to find their voices and contribute to this call for change, and do so with recommendations from the patient's perspective, to move toward a more patient-centered institution. The system must be transformed, doctors now say. They can facilitate that transformation by inviting and assisting this important feedback loop from their customers, the patients. This new awareness is a bit reminiscent of the way average folks have come to think about government. It is their government. It is there to serve them. They want and need to be heard. What is essential now has less to do with size and everything to do with effective performance and accountability. Who is really being served and how well? If we do this successfully, the patient-centered institution is headed our way.

Lost Future to "No Harm"

My summons to surgery following the irreparable harm inflicted during the first surgical encounter was frightening, heralded by intense abdominal pain and nausea that required an immediate emergency response. These debilitating attacks, so frequent and exhausting, given the time anticipated for recovery, curtailed virtually all normal activity and left me terribly weak and emotionally depressed. I faced immediate, emergency, same-day hospitalization and surgical preparation.

My wife and I became captives of my chronic incapacitating condition. This began in 2007, and the experience has been like living on the fault line of a tectonic plate or within reach of an active volcano. To this day, among my travel credentials, I continue to keep a medical folder updated and available. The extensive recreational pursuits we had planned have been virtually eliminated. We never know when the next crisis will strike—note, not *if* but *when*.

As my wife and I got older, we learned, as have most of you, to covet the rewards derived from hard work, well-deserved occasions for new and enriching experience. We have very high regard for a disciplined and deliberative life based on thoughtful planning— our small part of the American Dream. Optimistically, we assumed retirement would be very enjoyable. My wife and I were lucky enough to reside in a lovely college town, nationally known as one of the more admired and recognized, a real gem among communities and ideal for retirees. But fate, driven in large part by the system of concealment and medical incompetency, and compounded by equipment failures and faulty design, had a way of trumping even our most promising and sanguine possibilities and plans.

Medical Care Is in Your Future

Medical treatment is indispensable in all of our lives. It is time to echo the call initiated by some of our esteemed medical professionals. They have strongly asserted the urgent need for improvement. They insist on the penetrating light of transparency for the good of all patients, potential patients, hospitals, and members of the broader medical community as an incentive for change. My medical disclosure in the form of this careful, factual narrative is my contribution to this endeavor. A patient's perspective brings valuable insight into the consequences of medicine, performed well or gone terribly wrong. It inspires the hope that transparency, which is now regarded as that potent thrust toward accountability and becomes an antidote to medical unfairness and stagnation, will prevail. It is unbearable that patients are being endangered and killed with repeated systemic failures—the fact that this is happening in such unbelievable numbers is of the utmost importance for all of us. Since we have been inundated with the most benevolent and benign depictions of our medical services, I have chosen a dramatic scenario to awaken you to a more realistic portrait of the horrific casualties awaiting us absent dramatic systemic changes.

Chapter Three

A Hospital: The Most Dangerous Institution in the World

Silently Killing One Hundred Thousand per Year

As it turns out, hospitals are the most dangerous institutions in the world, places where killing is silent and mistakes are buried. According to a *New York Times* article by Dr. Sanjay Gupta,[9] it is actually difficult to determine how many fatalities occur annually, but the number could be up to two hundred thousand per year. Gupta goes on to explain that the very tests and procedures designed to protect doctors from malpractice lawsuits, what he calls "defensive medicine," can result in more deaths and injuries.

Abstract mortality beckons under the crushing weight of such statistics. These are astronomical numbers, but they represent real people—each and every one—and, when visibly portrayed, are shocking. Things going terribly wrong should be prevented whenever possible. My commitment is constructive and preventive. When we give voice to the victims of a system run amuck, these casualties of our mostly unintended perpetrators (which represent a horror nonetheless) can become a force for change.

What is it like to be the victim of a mistaken death sentence? A glimmer of hope is that some progressive medical leaders, who once

---

[9] Sanjay Gupta, "More Treatment, Less Mistakes," New York Times, July 14, 2012.

championed concealment for ostensibly legal and personal reasons, now regard concealing and burying mistakes as immoral and also destructive for the medical community. Unless tragic mistakes are fully vetted and understood, they are destined to be repeated.

Equivalent to Thirty 9/11s per Year

Graphically, hospital-inflicted loss of human life represents a stunning tragedy exceeding in mortality rate thirty 9/11 attacks annually. I am not making light of that devastation. But we have an ongoing calamity and the enemy is within—systemically. What I describe here has been alluded to quietly but consistently for decades. Total ferocity is precluded inasmuch as this tragedy occurs surreptitiously, with little recognition because it is so shrewdly camouflaged. Now medical professionals have begun to break ranks and are themselves denouncing the system that perpetuates such carnage. Many of them are taking on the system. Let's give credit where credit is due. Allow me another dramatic parallel.

Comparable to 330 Tragic Airline Crashes per Year

Envision an analogous disaster resulting from sequential airline crashes, each snuffing out the lives of three hundred or more passengers every day. To match our medical slaughter, this scenario would necessitate in excess of 330 crashes in any given year, roughly six per week—about one a day excluding the Sabbath.

Instant outrage and demand for action would erupt in under a week. If not addressed immediately, people would take to the streets in protest and stage an "Occupy Airports" movement. When graphically confronted, as a disastrous equivalent to a strikingly visible human tragedy that closely portrays a match in numbers, our quiet unobservable medical massacre is translated into a proportionate crisis that can no longer exist as an abstraction. We see it. We know it. It is undeniable. We are now forced to confront it. It is inevitable that we will know some victims, personally. A surprising number of exceptional medical representatives, who know it all too well, have sounded their alarm to confirm this. Stay with me, and I will call your attention to several of them. They could no longer remain silent.

Most Dangerous Institution in the World

Is a hospital the most dangerous institution in the world? Think I am being absurd? Look closer. This haunting statistic is so frequently reported: we quietly kill nearly one hundred thousand patients a year, and as we have seen, some medical experts believe the figure is twice that. If true, it brands hospitals—and this is not hyperbole—the most dangerous institutions in the world. The numbers confirm it, repeatedly. Let's pursue that presumably rash accusation. We're inundated with consoling images of hospitals and medical delivery systems as soothing, safe, and secure. The backdrop in presentations by pharmaceutical companies and high-tech medical equipment distributors depicts the hospital environment as the very antitheses of dangerous. But remember, hospitals are in the business of selling; and keep in mind, profits come first. We shall dissect the implications of that as well—it's the Wall Street connection.

Hospital Haven or Combat Zone?

As soon as you are admitted as a patient, you have been assigned to this perilous zone. It may be comparable to the hazards experienced on the frontlines of a raging battlefield. This comes as a result of mostly preventable medical errors found primarily in our hospitals; surgical infections, blood loss, anesthesia reactions, and prescription errors abound. Tired, overworked professionals, and on a lower level, insufficiently trained personnel, many working long hours at or near minimum wage, succumb to distraction, fatigue, and exhaustion.

This indictment is shocking. The terrifying number is incredible but seldom challenged. This is not an overstatement, no attempt to exaggerate. This is reality. That next whistling artillery shell, in the form of a virus, bacterium, medication mix-up, missed diagnosis, surgical error, or the like, may have your name on it—or that of your child, family member, or friend. It can be just as deadly as the shrapnel from a screeching, incoming shell. Staying with the military metaphor, this would constitute death from friendly fire or collateral damage. The grim notification will not come by cablegram but from a white-coated medical professional, attempting to put the best face on a horrible and preventable tragedy for which accountability is systematically denied.

Our life-saving medical institutions have an ominous reputation jolted by unbelievable data that keeps coming. The deaths from medical errors accompanied by a clandestine practice, decades old, of quietly burying mistakes, is most unsettling because it is the face of the problem. The figure looms large to the point of being incomprehensible were it not for having been cited repeatedly and remaining uncontested for many years. But now, insiders—doctors themselves—no longer willing to tolerate such atrocities on their watch, are coming forward in commendable numbers. As a knowledgeable patient, I'm happy to see it before more unwary patients are killed. One hundred thousand deaths each year: more than double the number of people killed in car crashes, five times the number killed in homicides, twenty times the total number of our armed forces killed in Iraq and Afghanistan.

The Transparency Solution

Fundamental issues regarding responsible regulation and the role of government in prevention and protection should be cultivated assertively. A bipartisan plan of action should be developed now to stave off the relentless carnage. This is strong language, but we have a crisis, which has been effectively, deliberately hidden from the American people. Professionals agree that comprehensive systemic changes are necessary. Committed leadership targeting practical, attainable goals is needed to move us forward. This cannot spontaneously evolve unaided from within our health care system. Effective incentives will be required, and it goes without saying, they could be stubbornly resisted in the profit-driven, greed-governed system that currently exists. A twist on the old adage is applicable: you can take the people out of the system, but it is more difficult to take the system out of the people. No Harm Street must be overhauled; too many are being harmed, and we have failed to learn from errors because that would require comprehensive disclosure, investigation, and acceptance of responsibility—yes, being held accountable. Alerts signaling the dangerous curves, dilapidated bridges, and visual blind spots that were primarily the result of inadequate regulations over decades, compounded by bad incentives, have brought us where we are today. The culture of concealment keeps us there. It must go. Transparency is a 180-degree pivot. Top medical professionals themselves recognize that nothing less will suffice.

Telling it like it is, from a patient's perspective, and striving for a level of disclosure rarely embraced in medicine or many other institutions can only help to enhance our most essential of all human services—the pursuit of health and wellness. Sharing my medical experience is my small contribution; it is the unvarnished truth of how I was helped and hurt, treated and mistreated. It will give voice to the hundreds of thousands who have suffered and continue to suffer in this system of secrecy. These unaddressed, hidden misfortunes exposed will benefit all when medical transparency prevails. The science of medicine has too long been burdened by this culture of concealment. "Burying mistakes" is a discomforting euphemism facing the profession that reflects its members' lack of openness. What becomes blatantly clear is this: it is not understated. Trust cannot emerge without concomitant verification, and that requires transparency.

This is not a witch hunt but a contribution for the improvement of our health care system. Our lives depend on it. I am telling the truth, so specific, critical, and unpleasant incidents are depicted in vivid detail while personal identities are protected. Countless victims, living and dead, and numerous dedicated servants at all levels comprising a reputable and thriving medical community, stand to benefit directly or indirectly. This is not for the patient alone but also for dedicated medical professionals who commit their lives to providing excellent medical treatment and embracing the ideals of that hallowed medical dictum, "First, do no harm!" Attention all medical professionals: you too will sooner or later become patients; you're improving a system that will ultimately save your lives as well—so climb aboard.

The Media Joins the Crusade

On April 28, 2013, the CBS News program *60 Minutes* carried the bizarre account of a serial killer working as a nurse in multiple New Jersey and Pennsylvania hospitals. He murdered an estimated forty patients by giving them toxic doses of medication. Their ages ranged from twenty-one to ninety-one, and his crimes spanned a period of sixteen years, involving seven different hospitals. These incidents of villainous behavior were accentuated by the paranoid culture of concealment run amok.

Charles Graeber documents this grizzly narration in his recent book *The Good Nurse*.[10] The story of nurse Charlie Cullen carves another notch in a bewildering institution that continues to sustain an appalling record for killing approximately one hundred thousand patients per year, most of which result from unintentional but preventable medical errors.

This account unveils a glaring weakness in the system, depicting personal and ethical lapses, and concealment as opposed to confrontation, even with patients' lives at stake. Has the profession established a grotesque record in providing Charles Cullen with an atrocious license to kill? I've heard very little regarding the medical administrators responsible for Cullen's employment being charged or brought to justice.

But here's an encouraging note: there are many inside the institution convinced that transparency will lead to better accountability. One of these professionals, Dr. Marty Makary, from Johns Hopkins, relates noteworthy episodes in his recent book, *Unaccountable: What Hospitals Won't Tell You and How Transparency Can Revolutionize*

---

[10] Charles Graeber, *The Good Nurse: A True Story of Medicine, Madness, and Murder* (New York: Twelve, 2013).

Health Care.[11] The implication derived from these recent disclosures is that it can be open season on patients—even at the hands of the mentally deranged. So, whether doing harm is accidental, intentional, or a form of outright incompetence, it's too frequent.

Dr. Makary readily confesses his own complicity in the concealment, which he defines as standard practice and which he and others are trying to change. One ineffectual surgeon, he noted as a new intern, had an earned reputation. He was dubbed Dr. HODAD. When Makary inquired, he was told the nickname stood for "Hands of Death and Destruction" because of the number of patients who had been victimized by his numerous botched surgeries.

His abbreviated message to the medical community regarding openness and accountability is that it can be resolved through transparency: "To do no harm going forward, we must be able to learn from the harm we have already done." Most everyone reading this book can cite experiences of outstanding and compassionate care received from the best institutions in our communities. We are delighted when that is our reality. But that is not always true everywhere and for everyone.

Learn from the Past or Repeat It

Our hope for the medical community is this: learn from your mistakes—don't repeat them. Out with the destructive and deeply entrenched culture of concealment that quietly but unquestionably kills repeatedly and incessantly. In return let's express support for the pursuit of medical transparency, which is beginning to gain momentum on several fronts. Our system needs reform. As patients,

---

[11] Makary, *Unaccountable.*

we can contribute to that reform by providing honest and relevant feedback in the proper setting.

Many medical professionals may have little appreciation of how things look from the patient's point of view. Even when they become patients themselves, these professionals may be so coddled and preferentially treated as insiders that their experience in the hospital setting may be drastically different from what the average person experiences. To that extent they cannot as easily identify with the experience of the typical patient. My contribution to the upcoming potential reform is to tell it like it has been for me without dissimulation. You are reading a living, uncensored, unconcealed account of my experience. What lends some credence to my report are the volcanic eruptions—confessions, if you will—from doctors themselves.

Secrecy Is a Costly Sacrifice

As my saga unfolded, I related pertinent experiences and discussions with medical professionals to gather support for future patients and for the medical community. Striving for a more insightful transparency is regarded as essential for attaining more successful performances, fewer complications, and more positive outcomes. I urge my readers to be aware that for most of my treatment, concealment appeared to be the ironclad, prearranged, albeit unspoken, order of the day.

It is most encouraging now that this posture, resulting in denial of responsibility, is being challenged and regarded as a systemic weakness rather than a strength. Originally designed to protect the system, at least ostensibly, the culture of concealment is currently regarded as an impediment, detrimental to medical progress. Now it appears that influential elements of the medical community regard transparency as essential to enhancing performance. Institutional protection via concealment is counterproductive—it precludes medical progress.

Dr. No Show

My narrative will at times portray the emotions I experienced accompanied by the corresponding behaviors to which I am responding through this book. You are therefore free to conclude whether it's balanced or excessive. Since it is my genuine personal experience, you will see emotion in my presentation. Emotion is a part of life, so I won't pretend to be detached, though with hindsight I have stepped back to assure my overall objectivity. You will encounter and evaluate my surgeon, who performed the robot-assisted procedure that resulted in my life-altering medical complications. I am being very candid since this resulted in the series of events central to this book. I am trying to be as accurate as possible in sharing the encounters prior to, during, and following the actual surgical encounter. This narrative in retrospect portrays the doctor as I came to perceive him. He performed that critical first surgery, bringing on the series of medical crises that radically diminished my life and health. His dismissive unreliability, evidenced before the first surgery and during the follow-up, was both revealing and bizarre, a noteworthy example of a behavior pattern you will wish to avoid (and I hope you succeed).

These medical incongruities depict several scenarios I now regard as irresponsible. I was totally unprepared for the uncanny arena I was thrust into. In a very real sense I happened to be in the wrong place at the wrong time, and the result was disaster. The cloak of medically sanctioned approval should not be taken at face value as quality assured, as you will see as you come to understand the role of concealment within the system. My experience under this surgeon's care resulted in the necessity of five (and counting) subsequent serious abdominal surgeries in as many years. These successive surgeries were readily conceded to stem from a severe medical complication during the first procedure, performed robotically, to remove a contained cancerous prostate. The complications that followed and the botched attempts to repair the damage resulted in a life-threatening hematoma that left me on the verge of death for several weeks.

Our First Encounter

I met my doctor—a surgeon whom I can only describe as robotic—for the very first time in midsummer 2007 and elected to have him perform my prostate biopsy. He appeared to have superior credentials, a part of which was an internship at one of the finest hospitals in the country. The quantity of procedures performed was adequate to quell any doubt about his experiential competency. At this time he was introducing a technique that allowed the visualization of the prostate as he took a series of biopsied samples that would enhance the diagnostic potential. I was relieved to be having the process completed since I had been prepped twice before and appeared for my appointment at the urologic center only to be told the doctor would not be available. On the first occasion a conflict in appointments was cited, and the second time he demurred, indicating that he was experiencing severe back pain and would need to reschedule. It seems to me that, both times, courtesy would have dictated that he contact me prior to the time I showed up and was prepped for the appointment. This type of courtesy should be protocol, since that type of runaround is a significant inconvenience for a patient. In hindsight, I can see that should have been a yellow caution flag. I missed a vital signal—don't you!

My error: I held a naïve, misplaced trust in the medical system, expecting it to maintain a standard quality of performance for service to patients. I was in for a rude awakening. That did not exist in the medical community and does not now exist according to disclosures from many highly respected medical professionals. No one appeared to be in charge. We were encountering a professional who seemed not to be in charge of himself. Many, it seemed, did pretty much as they pleased. That, to my dismay, proved to be the medical norm, but you be the judge as you read, listen, observe, and learn. One lesson to learn from this is that if the doctor you are working with does not behave in a professional manner, find another, if possible.

Biopsy in 3-D

The procedure I elected was called a transrectal 3-D ultrasound guided biopsy. A group of a half-dozen residents and seasoned professionals were assembled to witness the new technique. The room, well equipped and superbly lighted, was normally used for cosmetic surgery. The mood was jovial, a popcorn atmosphere. We jested about the possible enhancing potential this new technology might bring about: Given the proclivity for creative billing that had been reported recently, one might even be charged for a twofold augmentation! The medical community might mull that over.

The humor relieved tension as I lay splayed in the presence of this group of men and women. Each biopsy was extracted by an accompanying distinctive pop resembling the discharge of a muffled cap pistol firing. There was also a sharp, painful stinging sensation lasting a few seconds with each. If memory serves me, sixteen such probes were made and as many biopsy samples extracted. The entire procedure took less than an hour.

Awaiting test results on serious health issues usually leaves most of us understandably anxious. I was notified on a Friday that I should come in Monday to discuss some concerns with my biopsy. As a patient and since the doctor had alluded to obvious concerns, I felt that weekend stretch into an eternity. Having experienced this, I would not knowingly subject a patient to that prolonged wait. The medical community should address this issue if possible. And from the patient's perspective, this appears to reflect a lack of empathy he would not wish on himself or his relatives. Therein lies the compassionate criterion for caring. I am going to call it the Golden Rule applied to medicine and life. I will expand on this later without apology. This would encourage medical professionals to structure their communications in ways that would reduce tension, without misrepresentation to others, as much as possible.

The Diagnosis

Again I call upon my medical record while protecting the identity of specific professionals and institutions.

> July 2007, Mr. Huber had a recent biopsy of the prostate performed by [my robotic surgeon] . . . as a result of his elevated PSA in the free PSA. He was found to have one focus of Gleason score 6 prostate cancer, very small volume disease, however located in the apex of the prostate. He came here to discuss the findings today. The patient is well read and very well informed.

We have discussed all the options of treatment of prostate cancer including watchful waiting, different types of radiation therapy, and different types of surgery. The patient is interested to get a second opinion as far as pathology is concerned and also will discuss this issue with the radiation oncologist. He is inclined to have robotic surgery, however, and I have reassured him that [this hospital,] at the present time, is one of the best places in the country to have it done. Mr. Huber will contact me the moment he makes the final decision. . . .

The above was written by an internationally renowned surgeon (not my robotic surgeon), a professor at the college of medicine in the department of urology. Following confirmation of the pathology diagnosis, we scheduled the surgery.

Chapter Four

First Surgery

The Big Day: Complications

My robotic surgeon returned from a trip abroad a day prior to my surgery. The morning of the surgery, he called expressing some concern, saying he had just acquainted himself with my blood profile, a routine procedure for all pending surgeries. It had been available for two weeks. For several years I've been troubled by chronic anemia, which the report reflected, and he wished to consult with my hematologist to determine whether he was supportive of the imminent surgery planned for that afternoon. My hematologist had monitored my stable condition for a few years and was supportive of the surgery.

Routine hospital delays prevented our starting until early evening. The anticipated duration was four hours, barring complications. The use of the term *complications*—what hospitals and doctors alike do not wish to disclose and are uncomfortable discussing—reflects a lack of transparency that is a systemic weakness. We had complications, multiple complications, cascading to an irreparable life-threatening and life-altering outcome in a short period of time.

Certain procedures went terribly wrong, which I will recount. I reference my abbreviated, medical record for the benefit of interested professionals and inquiring laypersons. The more casual reader may wish to pass over these technical insertions, which spell out in medicalese the actual procedures. My purpose is to disclose what occurred. I share the account from the surgeon's perspective as posted in my record. The medical community is now beginning to appreciate the potential role of transparency for our and their understanding and security. It appears that this issue is now being spearheaded by the medical profession. This has become especially pertinent to the reduction of concealment. And that in turn is regarded as advancing the medical profession, as its members become more serious about learning from rather than concealing medical mistakes. Had transparency prevailed, I would not now be guessing about what really transpired during my robotic surgery. The reader may further appreciate my aroused interest with the quite sudden media coverage of the da Vinci robotic surgery that follows.

Robotic Trauma

The day I met da Vinci, I survived robotic surgery of the prostate— barely. I quote my medical record to establish the credibility of my narrative and specify the remarkable similarities with the more recent allegations surrounding this robotic device on some procedures from the multiple media sources now flooding the airwaves. Numerous legal charges have been leveled against the manufacturer and various surgeons. These discoveries were not available when I had the surgery as reported below.

> The Operative Report, 11-19-07 is instructive. [I am abbreviating, to avoid redundancy.]
> Operation Performed: Robotic radical prostatectomy with bilateral partial nerve-sparing using hemostatic hydrodissector and repair of rectal injury with consultation intraoperatively with Trauma Surgery [*This was addressing*

*the restoration of the accidental rectal injury that resulted
in subsequent potentially lethal infections*] . . . repair the
defect in two layers using 2-0 silk sutures in interrupted
fashion and then Lembert sutures.

This was performed and a repeat rectal exam revealed
the defect had been corrected. . . . The left robotic arm was
inspected. [*Was that arm not performing properly, or did
they lack essential skills—or both?*] There appeared to be a
slight injury to the epigastric vessels and therefore Carter-
Thompson suture was used to suture ligate these vessels.
No bleeding was noted thereafter. . . . Complications:
Rectal injury as mentioned above with rectal repair.

The robotic arm or the pilots appear to have gone off course—
perhaps both? It may be revealing to see a random review of surgical
reports on da Vinci, focusing on the robotic arms, while protecting
the identity of the patients. Is the arm evaluated when a surgery
appears to have proceeded without complications? Or do we find this
explanation mentioned only when the outcome is suspect?

When your favorite baseball team is in a close game and the
pitcher, who has up to that point found the strike zone with effective
regularity, suddenly finds himself walking several batters, the outcome
is jeopardized. The trainer is called out, not when the pitcher is doing
well, but when he is performing poorly. This may not be the perfect
parallel, but you get the point. Why check the robotic arm? A patient's
life may never be the same as a result of a surgery if something goes
terribly wrong. A current report on da Vinci appeared recently in the
Wall Street Journal.[12]

12 Joseph Walker, "Intuitive Surgical Warns of Problem With Robot Tool:
Instruments Used in Robots Can Momentarily Stall During Procedures, FDA
Advises," *Wall Street Journal*, December 4, 2013.

In this article, the company that manufactures da Vinci robotic equipment, Intuitive Surgical, admitted that the robotic arm could stall during surgical procedures: "The company said that friction within instrument arms can interrupt the instruments' motion, according to a notice posted on the FDA's website."

We may never know for certain who holds responsibility for failure; again, concealment is operating here. Irreparable damage was done, and in the absence of accountability, as usual, the patient sustained the full costs of pain, suffering, and loss for this tragic outcome. The medical community is actually paid for errors, rewarded exponentially, since each subsequent procedure is fully charged to the patient. Even if performed incorrectly, when repeated, it is charged again! If the patient dies, bury the mistakes! Unfortunately with that stratagem, little learning takes place.

Did the trauma center possess the requisite robotic experience to assist effectively? This is a valid question that is raised by implication frequently in the recent media attention received by da Vinci. Many of the symptoms disclosed in my operational report coincide closely with the recently revealed malfunctions reported repeatedly with the da Vinci procedures.

Recent reports have described many damaging events:

- A robotic hysterectomy procedure in 2012 resulted in the death of a woman when a blood vessel was nicked.

- A New York man's colon was pierced during prostate surgery.

- A robotic arm vice-gripped tissue during colorectal surgery in January of 2013. The total system had to be shut down in order to release the jaws. That report indicated the patient was not seriously injured.

- A robotic arm struck the patient in the face during a hysterectomy procedure. The surgeon discontinued use of the robot and finished with conventional surgery.

Intuitive Surgical (the manufacturer) was the source for most of these accidents.

Several class-action lawsuits have been filed as a result of the robotic surgeries, and examples of the charges include:

- Peritonitis: inflammation of the lining of the abdomen
- Sepsis: widespread infection
- Excessive bleeding
- Burning of nearby organs, including the intestines
- Punctured blood vessels, organs, and arteries
- Severe bowel injuries
- Punctured or cut ureters

Adding to the controversy, CNBC[13] carried a series in April 2013 in a debate format that represented most interested parties. In a related article, reporter Herb Greenberg wrote:
According to lawsuits, complaints, interviews with alleged victims, plaintiff attorneys and a database, many of the reported injuries during robotic surgery appear to be burns and other heat-related damage to intestines, ureter, bowels and other organs.

---

[13] Herb Greenberg, "Part 1, Controversy Over Surgical Robotics Heats Up, Retrieved from http://www.cnbc.com/id/100650872," CNBC, April 18, 2013; Herb Greenberg "Part 2: Patients Scarred After Robotic Surgery," *CNBC*, April 19, 2013; Herb Greenberg "Part 3: Counting the Problems of Robot-Assisted Surgery," *CNBC*, April 19, 2013; Herb Greenberg "Part 4: Marketing Is Key to Surgical Robot's Success," *CNBC*, April 19. 2013.

Medical Madness

My own personal experience cost me my health and nearly my life. Naturally, it has made me more than an inquisitive spectator. It gave voice to my intuitive perception of the relationship between my symptoms and the medical realities disclosed. I believe—but cannot prove—that injuries were purposely hidden from me at the time of my surgery; that would not be inconsistent with the longstanding medical practice of concealment. The injuries were severe, but given the concealment posture and the contractual protection afforded the institution treating me, I found it virtually impossible to get legal representation. My family and I were left to carry the burden and loss alone.

Nevertheless, the disclosure of legal challenges was a vindication of sorts. Even with the current multiple invitations to join legal pursuits, I have chosen not to participate, given the statute of limitations in my case. I am encouraged to see others go forward since this seems to be one way to bring about safer procedures for future patients. Rewarding tragic surgical outcomes financially by allowing hospitals to bill for their mistakes will only tend to duplicate inferior performances. At the same time, I encourage readers to be cognizant of newly reported da Vinci malfunctions.

The attempted repair of the injury I suffered during this first surgery resulted in a potentially fatal infection. The devastation that followed raised troubling questions—but brought no answers. Fact: the repair proved inadequate. (The rupture of the ligate, as reported, resulted in life-threatening infections, adding credence to this assumption). The no-harm philosophy here seems mythical. Medical professionals appear to lack the rigorous incentives, professional and ethical, for encouraging optimal disclosure. Accountability is not assigned. The patient bears the burden. Accountability—acceptance of responsibility for errors and for any resultant harm—is missing.

Expense and career implications based on evaluated performance should bring about a decidedly more responsible outcome.

So consider this a call for accountability: Robotic performance required a substantial period of training including regular practice to maintain the requisite skills. If trauma's assistance was a part of the solution, absent adequate robotic training, do they not share accountability for contributing to a faulty procedure to rectify the injury sustained in the complications? The robotic system, at the time, was relatively new to this institution, though it was introduced to the broader medical community in 2000, ushering in the new millennium.

Robotic inexperience is cited increasingly as a reason for injuries to patients. Professionals have attempted to assist, absent sufficient robotic skills, to collaborate in a vital task in an unpracticed setting and with a need to perform to near perfection; outcomes may indicate they have not yet mastered essential procedures. The results have the earmarks of inadequate skills. Concealment still covers many medical errors, and untested and unreliable improvising can be the order of the day.

In my own case, several things went dreadfully wrong. The attempted repair resulted in further complications, which I must allow the record drafted from the surgeons' viewpoint to recount [though I have little reason to fully trust it given concealment's dominance in medical practice]. Putting the best face on an aberrant outcome seems to be routine. Again, the casual reader may wish to pass over these technical narratives, which spell out in medicalese the precise encounters, procedures, and repercussions recorded that fateful night. They make for laborious reading, except for medical professionals, but reviewing them is necessary for those wishing to establish, professionally, the quality of the performance. Some may feel that, inasmuch as this is personal, since the event reduced my ability to do the things I loved, I may have a tendency to exaggerate; this is not the case. In fact, I wish to point out that it appears questions I raised in 2007 have been vindicated as we view cumulative records appearing in 2013. I have garnered a great deal of company; rest assured my empathy is with them.

Renegade Robots?

First, let me cite the Associated Press, which raised serious questions about robotic surgery in April 2013.

> The biggest thing in operating rooms these days is a million-dollar, multi-armed robot named da Vinci, used in nearly 400,000 surgeries nationwide last year—triple the number just four years earlier.
> But now the high-tech helper is under scrutiny over reports of problems, including several deaths that may be linked with it, and the high cost of using the robotic system. There also have been a few disturbing, freak incidents:
> During surgery a robotic arm hit a patient in the face as she lay on the operating table.
> A robotic hand that wouldn't let go of tissue grasped.
> Is it time to curb the robot enthusiasm?[14]

In a another article, author Lindsey Tanner reported on "a robotic arm that wouldn't let go of tissue grasped during colorectal surgery on Jan. 14. 2012. 'We had to do a total system shutdown to get the grasper to open its jaws,' claimed the report filed by the hospital. The report also said the patient was not injured."

---

[14] Associated Press, "Surgical Robot da Vinci Scrutinized by FDA after Deaths, Other Surgical Nightmares," *New York Daily News*, April 9, 2013.

Tanner added that "an upcoming research paper suggests that problems linked with robotic surgery are underreported."[15]

The robotic surgery malfunctions include cases with "catastrophic complications," according to Dr. Marty Makary, whom you met earlier championing transparency. Dr. Makary is himself an experienced robotic surgeon, so his commentary on da Vinci may be given requisite credence.

The list of concerns is formidable. This robot is aptly named given its conspicuous incursion into avant-garde medical technology. Our celebrated artist, Leonardo da Vinci, helped define the Italian Renaissance, living from 1452 to 1519. Da Vinci was one of the most brilliant men of his generation and arguably one of the brightest who ever lived. He ranks among the world's greatest painters and sculptors and has received glowing accolades for his work as an architect, engineer, mathematician, and inventor. His great art included most popularly the paintings *Mona Lisa* and *The Last Supper.*

Time magazine[16] charted the ways that technology has impacted our lives. Our recent incursion into robotics and corollaries includes artificial intelligence, notably IBM's Watson computer (used on the TV game show *Jeopardy*), chess-playing computers used in several more progressive nations, industrial manufacturing models, a robotic automobile, and more. The variety and complexity of current technology have become mythical—invading, aiding and abetting us in our fictional fantasies and beyond. In his article, David Von Drehle notes the shipping crane, welding robot, airline kiosk, surgical

---

[15] Lindsey Tanner. "Robot Hot among Surgeons but FDA Taking Fresh Look," *Associated Press*. April 13, 2013. http://bigstory.ap.org/article/robot-hot-among-surgeons-fda-taking-new-look.

[16] David Von Drehle, "Winners and Losers in the New Robot Economy," *Time*, September 9, 2013.

robot, Roomba (used to vacuum our floors), warehouse bot, disaster responders, and driverless car.

The impact of robotics on Wall Street, Main Street, and No Harm Street is immeasurable and growing exponentially. Robots have taken us captive, and we haven't yet seen the half of it. The influence on politics, policy, personal and medical systems, and the economy are cited. There are no projected villains; systems dominate behavior. Robotics represent a system too, and consequently sparks will fly. The novelist is in charge of his creation—the theme, characters, setting, and so on. We create and command; the brighter we are, the more brilliant the robotic characters. The plot defines what the robot does. When they/we kill ourselves through our own creation, it is tragic, and we want to shift the responsibility. But we are accountable; these results overrule our objections for responsibility. We are accountable for our robots. They may periodically rebel, through our programming errors or design flaws, but we are their creators; we rule, and we are responsible.

The da Vinci experience brings to mind classics of science fiction, such as Stanley Kubrick's 1968 film *2001: A Space Odyssey,* which represents the problems of robotic intelligence. As Hal, the lifelike robotic intelligence piloting the space vehicle begins to digress from the planned destination (or malfunctions, if you prefer), his human counterparts were unable to control him. Hal is disturbing in ominous ways. When the crew resists his deviation from expectations, he begins killing humans with impunity. He justifiably feels threatened by their plot to dissect his circuitry and virtually eliminate him. It is the classic survival-of-the-fittest scenario, with numerous casualties. Hal is finally shut down as his modules are removed one by one, his incoherence depicted as he resonates vocally, weakly echoing both his resistance and demise. Recall that in one of the previously mentioned articles, our celebrated surgical robot had to be de-energized to render it inert and release vice-gripped tissue and pinned-down patients as the symbolic hostility played out. Revisit either the novel or the movie version of *2001: A Space Odyssey*—they are classics and have never been more current or relevant than now. Potential here is a double-edged sword.

In the medical encounters with da Vinci, the eerie parallels are arresting as we look at specific afflictions resulting from encounters with surgical patients. The FDA attempts to reign in the risks by tracking the outcomes to make sure that humans have firmer control of the consequences and that, when evaluated objectively to assure accountability, devices meet verifiable standards of acceptability.

A series of reports from leading media sources focused on the increasing use of da Vinci robotic surgeries and raised questions concerning their safety, functional appropriateness, economy (e.g., profits over patients), and the experience and competency of surgeons using the da Vinci. The FDA is investigating the use and performance of robotic surgery instruments given the growing adoption of the technology and the apparent resulting increase in complications. A *New York Times* article refers disturbingly to the "salesmen in the surgical suite"[17] and describes how the major manufacturer of the da Vinci surgical equipment, Intuitive Surgical, encouraged minimal training for hospital personnel while encouraging unlimited sales of their systems—a short term high and long term disaster.

My interest in the new disclosures was spiked because my experience was life-altering and began with a da Vinci surgical procedure. In this book, I've shared the encounter I had with the

---

[17] Roni Caryn Rabini, "Salesmen in the Surgical Suite," *New York Times*, March 26, 2013.

robot that appears to have been partially responsible for my need for a series of additional follow-up surgeries resulting in the horrific decline in my own physical health. I took the liberty of responding to the invitation for comments in the *Wall Street Journal*'s article by Christopher Weaver and Joseph Walker, published February 28, 2013, "The FDA Seeks Data on Surgical Robots." I was quoted in the comments section of the article summarizing my experience, hoping the FDA would notice and consider patients' input as well.

Using the medical report which I quoted earlier in this book, I explained my own experience with the da Vinci robotic system and added:

> I have had four subsequent surgeries to repair the damage incurred as a result of the complications from that robotic encounter. I was a healthy, athletic 75 year old male. In a month I dropped from 145 lbs. to 110, barely clinging to life as a result of the complications e.g., rectal injury and failed repair, hematoma, MRSA and adhesions. It ruined my life—health wise. I believe there is room for improvement in the use of this new technology.

The spate of media coverage seems to me to be long overdue.

I have referenced three articles briefly covering specific issues as well as an April 2013 report on CNBC. According to Herb Greenberg's 2013 review on CNBC:[18]

> The closest to a central database for medical device "adverse events" is the Food and Drug Administration's Manufacturer and User Facility Device Experience—or MAUDE—database.
>
> Since 2000, the database recounts reports of at least 85 deaths and 245 injuries related to Intuitive Surgical's da Vinci-related injuries.

---

18   Greenberg, "Counting the Problems."

During the same period, roughly 1.5 million robotic procedures have been performed. While some would argue that any death or injury could and should be unacceptable, the simple math suggests that reported problems are statistically insignificant in terms of overall risk.

Listed among the injuries are surgical burns to arteries or organs, peritonitis (painful inflammation of the lining of the abdomen), sepsis, excessive bleeding, burning of nearby organs including the intestines, punctured blood vessels of organs or arteries, burns, and/or tears of the intestines and other severe bowel injuries.

The *Wall Street Journal* explains that the da Vinci equipment can malfunction and may cause serious internal injury: "The latest issue affects nearly 1,400 instruments world-wide, though the number of affected robots is likely to be lower because some robots have more than one instrument, according to the company." [19]

Intuitive Surgical has sold more than 2,585 da Vinci systems worldwide. The company issued the warning about defective equipment after receiving three reports from customers, said David Rosa, senior vice president of scientific affairs, in an interview.

The company said that "friction within the instrument's arms can interrupt the instruments' motion," according to a notice posted on the FDA's website.

The cumulative descriptions of complications add more weight to the analysis of my 2007 surgery's outcome. The ensuing surgeries and life-altering diminished functioning that resulted may be related

---

[19]   Walker, Joseph. "Intuitive Surgical Warns of Problem with Robot Tool: Instruments Used in Robots Can Momentarily Stall During Procedures, FDA Advises." *Wall Street Journal*, December 4, 2013. http://online.wsj.com/news/article_email/SB10001424052702304451904579238182142888184-lMyQjAxMTAzMDAwNTEwNDUyWj.

to that difficult, robotically assisted surgery. The call for transparency by members of the medical community is relevant. Had that existed in my case, it would have made this a moot issue. I would now know; concealing such an event would have been virtually impossible.

Incentive Guidance

Hospitals perform poorly yet make more money. It is worth noting here as reported from current research that more money is often paid for poor performances. This obviously disturbing pattern of the absence of accountability results when a mistake is made and patients are charged repeatedly. Hospitals continue to demand payment, thus accepting no responsibility for poor performance. Since they practice within a culture of concealment, they seldom accept accountability for complications, even when it is so evident that it cannot be denied.

In a recent *Wall Street Journal* article,[20] Christopher Weaver highlights this point:

> Treatment complications and infections can inadvertently bolster the bottom line. Surgical complications such as infections and procedure-related strokes were on average twice as lucrative as operations that went smoothly at one large hospital system, researchers from Harvard Medical School, Boston Consulting Group and Texas Health Resources, reported Tuesday in the Journal of the American Medical Association.
>
> The new research found private-insurance and Medicare payments soared when surgeries went awry, outpacing extra treatment costs. In one example, a complication during an intestinal surgery performed on a Medicare patient could lead to an extended intensive-care stay, boosting payments fivefold.

---

[20]   Christopher Weaver, "Treatment Woes Can Bolster Profit," *Wall Street Journal,* April 17, 2013.

Chapter Five

Get It Right—Be Accountable

Silent routine killing can no longer be tolerated; it is hideous and unthinkable, yet it is a part of our system. Ironically the "no harm" mantra continues to mask accountability. It is a systemic smoke screen for unimaginable harm. The discharge summary from my 2007 surgery reads, in part:

> He was slowly advanced to a clear liquid diet and finally a full regular diet prior to discharge. The patient's hospital course was otherwise unremarkable. He did have a drain that was left in place in the pelvic fossa. His Foley catheter was also kept in place. He was discharged to home on antibiotics.

I remained hospitalized until November 24, 2007. Though the original expectation for the length of my hospital stay was overnight, my stay extended to five days.

A Gift of Infection and Too Busy to Bother

Not only was the original surgery marred by complications, but the surgeon's follow-up seemed irresponsible. The doctor's disinterest was apparent and accompanied by reckless decision making that exposed his patient (me) to a serious, growing infection. His medical judgment was seriously flawed. On my first return visit December 4, 2007, my surgeon removed a drain from my abdomen. I literally collapsed from the paralyzing pain. The surgeon assured my wife, as I lay curled in a fetal position on the examination table that he was confident it was nothing to be concerned with. He seemed to treat our apprehension and my condition as annoyances. He was obviously distracted and inattentive as he moved on to what was presumably his next appointment, literally leaving my life in jeopardy. He allowed a few moments for recuperation and then dismissed me to home.

As I arose from the table, I fainted, and with my wife's assistance, I was lowered to the floor. The surgeon returned, at my wife's request, and he returned me to the table. We remained briefly while my blood pressure was monitored, and then again I was released. I should not have been sent home with these alarming symptoms. Immediate intervention at that time might have mitigated the increasing infection developing within. I was confronted with that recurring tragic indifference on multiple occasions.

I regretted that I had not seriously regarded the evidence from my earliest impressions of my surgeon. The missed appointments and his tardy assessment of vital presurgical information early on were noteworthy. Now alarming evidence of postsurgical infection was obvious but discounted. Time was of the essence as the infection advanced. Most medical professionals would have seen a red flag in these symptoms and checked further—infections don't call time out.

My son commented in retrospect, "Dad, that is not the type of treatment he would have tolerated for his own father." A natural reference to our Golden Rule—what a difference that would make. The antibiotics were of little use; the infection soared, and my fever and pain mounted. My life was now in grave danger. We charted a hasty return to the hospital. The irreparable damage cited above had fueled the infection with a momentum that often kills. I was forced to return to the hospital on December 6, 2007, where I spent most of the month with what proved to be an overwhelming infection. Time and antibiotics, our only allies, came too little and almost too late. The raging enemy within—infection fueled by MRSA—had been surrendered to by our negligent surgeon's indifference. For those not familiar with this term, MRSA (methicillin-resistant *Staphylococcus aureus*) is a bacterium that has been responsible for many serious infections. The bacterium is highly resistant to modern drug treatment and as a result can be deadly. A fever in a case such as mine could easily represent a new MRSA progression.

The consultation report from December 8, 2007, read as follows:

Patient with a recent history of prostatectomy now with MRSA [bacteremia is an invasion of the bloodstream by bacteria] and questions of antibiotic management. The patient started developing abdominal pain, nausea and vomiting. He was seen by Urology as an outpatient on 12/04/07 at which time his Foley was removed as well as a drainage catheter from the operative site. A day prior to admission the patient had a temperature of 101.4 with worsening abdominal pain and was admitted on 12/06/07. . . . Urine cultures grew 10,000 to 100,000 mixed Gram-positive flora. Blood cultures from admission on 12/06/07, 2/2 sets were positive for MRSA. On 12/06/07 he had a chest x-ray which showed decreased lung volumes, no obvious consolidations and multiple distended bowel loops under the diaphragm. CAT scan of chest, abdomen and pelvis with contrast showed dilated small bowel loops, partial collapse of distal small bowel and colon consistent with partial SBO. There was a 7.3 x 4.2 cm fluid collection/abscess in the prostatic bed.

Bad Incentives—and Moral Hazards

Keep in mind I was examined by the surgeon on December 4, 2007, and experienced excruciating pain in his presence. At that time, he assured us it was nothing to be concerned about, yet two days later, on December 6, 2007, I returned to the hospital with a potentially lethal infection.

The doctor had no valid reason for his behavior. My record spells out the cost of his hurriedness and bad judgment. He was nevertheless rewarded (incentivized) to behave as he did. For him and the medical community, this was business as usual—more work, more experience for interns, more money from me for the medical establishment. The seriousness of his error, as usual, was never addressed openly by the medical community. Its members are consistent with their tradition, remaining nondisclosing and unaccountable. As countless patients will confirm—and I have lots of company—this is their SOP (standard operating procedure). I am writing this for all patients, about all patients, and for and about the medical community, who will themselves become patients—they too will benefit from an improved quality of service.

Second Surgery: Post–Da Vinci Encounter

Impression: Mr. Huber has developed MRSA bacteremia [the presence of bacteria in the blood. The blood is normally a sterile environment, so the detection of bacteria in the blood is always abnormal.] Secondary to postop wound infection in the prostate bed and this was presumed to be an abscess under pressure.

Recommendations: (1) To assure defervescence [return to normal body temperature after high fever] and prevent relapse, favor drainage of the prostatic bed abscess. (2) Continue antibiotics . . . (3) Check vancomycin trough. . . .

It was the consensus of the medical team that my condition now required major surgery to counter these life-threatening infections resulting from complications—their failures—from the original robotic surgery with rectal injury and the disastrous repair and follow-up by a negligent surgeon.

Preoperative Diagnosis: 12/12/2007 Small bowel obstruction.

Postoperative Diagnosis: (1) Pelvic phlegmon/hematoma [this is a spreading inflammatory process with formation of suppurative/purulent exudate or pus]. (2) High-grade partial and small and large bowel obstructions. (3) Appendicitis.

Findings: (1) A liquefied pelvic hematoma was found in proximity to the previous urologic surgery. (2) Adhesions between the small bowel and phlegmon, and sigmoid colon phlegmon, [*spreading inflammatory process and formation purulent exudate or pus*] led to apparent high-grade partial obstructions.

Description of Proceedure: . . . A Bookwalter retractor was placed to facilitate visualization. Dilated proximal small bowel led to the pelvic phlegmon. Electrocautery and blunt adhesiolysis was performed to release the small bowel and thus the obstruction. A loop of sigmoid colon was similarly adhesed to the inflammatory phlegmon, with proximal dilated colon. This was similarly released with blunt and electrocautery adhesiolysis. A liquefied pelvic hematoma was then drained. . . . Because the colon was distended, thus making abdominal closure more difficult, and because of the periappendicitis with the potential for frank appendicitis with further kinking of the appendix, an appendectomy was performed. With colonic decompression using a 14-French Retrovert Robinson catheter. . . . The abdomen was irrigated with saline, and homeostasis confirmed. . . . The suprapubic tube and drains placed by Urology were then sutured to the skin with multiple 2-0 Nylon sutures.

Continuing with details from my medical record, here is an assessment of my condition as of December 19, 2007:

Eval Source of Infection FINDINGS: The patient's bowel obstruction has been resolved post adhesiolysis [the surgical lysis, destruction or decomposition of adhesions]. There are 2 JP drains noted coursing through the anterior pelvis and terminating in the low pelvis. A Foley catheter and suprapubic catheter are also noted. There is a small amount of free intraperitoneal fluid that layers in the posterior pelvis which is not being drained by the surgical drains. In addition, there is approximately 5.8 × 5.1 cm collection of air and fluid located adjacent and superior portion of the bladder which may represent air and fluid within the superior portion of the bladder that is not being drained by the catheters, or may be a loculated [divided into small cavities or compartments] collection of fluid in the pelvis. This may be confirmed by instilling contrast through either the Foley or suprapubic catheters.

Clinging to Life—Refusing to Die

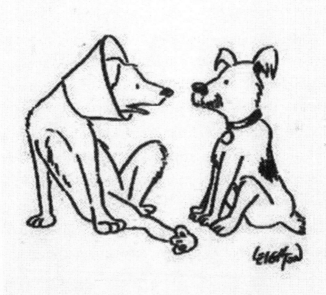

"I feel that I've been given a unique opportunity to speak out on the issues."

As we have seen from the recent da Vinci challenges, my experience is hardly coincidental. I have joined the group of casualties. This surgical procedure with complications resulted in life-endangering infections, a hematoma, MRSA, a couple of months (cumulatively) of hospital stays, with a perilously emaciated physical appearance. Recurring adhesions from this medical misadventure resulted in five (and counting) emergency bowel surgeries. And all of this was the result of a serious but routine surgical procedure, one that, if performed poorly—as my case reflects—can have disastrous consequences, and can even cause death.

"I'm Outta Here"

A close friend and tennis buddy of several years had a biopsy revealing a prostate malignancy in the same hospital and at approximately the same time I was being treated. He had considered having surgery there. Visiting me, following my procedure, and witnessing the complications in my tragic outcome—the hematoma, exacerbated by a MRSA infection, the near forty-pound weight loss in less than a month, and other related medical issues—blew his mind. He arranged immediately for his procedure to be performed at one of the nation's premier surgical institutions, where he had connections. He experienced an excellent outcome with no complications, utilizing the identical robotic procedure. With a similar diagnosis, different hospital, different surgeon, different patient, and similar surgical procedure, he experienced a highly successful outcome.

Chapter Six

Forever Healing, a Year and Counting

Wound Care Experience

My second hospital stay was terminated on December 26, 2007, and left me immobile and incapable of sitting up in bed unassisted. I was transferred to a local healthcare facility for recuperation. While there, I recovered sufficiently for tentative use of toilet facilities and learned to move about warily with the assistance of a walker. I exited on January 4, 2008 and was assisted by my wife at our residence.

No sooner had I learned my way around my home again than I experienced another attack of bowel obstruction. I return to my medical record.

01/07/08 Admission Date: Principal Diagnosis: Ileus [commonly defined simply as bowel obstruction] narcotic induced, versus partial small bowel obstruction.

Hospital Course: The patient presented to the emergency room with complaints of nausea, vomiting, having no bowel movement. A CT of the abdomen showed the partial small bowel versus ileus that was believed to be narcotic induced. . . . They evaluated the patient and felt that this was more ileus narcotic induced, felt that it was best to keep the patient NPO NG tube and monitor him closely. . . . NG tube was continued. . . . On 01/08/08 we had a PICC line placed for potential TPN and IV fluids since the patient was quite dehydrated on his admission. . . . The patient started having flatus on 01/09/08. The NG tube was again discontinued on 01/11/08. . . . The electrolytes were monitored. . . . On 01/12/08 the patient received a clear liquid diet. 01/16/08 the patient felt strong enough to be discharged home. . . . He had two JP drains. . . . The patient was slowly advanced to a soft diet by 01/14/08. . . . [D]rains in place since his surgery and were continuing to put out amounts higher than we felt comfortable removing.

My New Normal

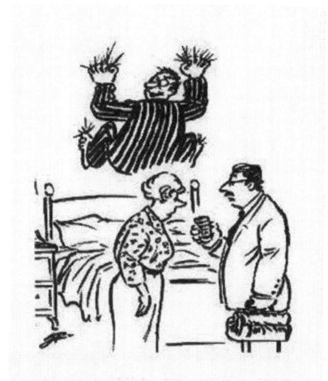

"I think I've found the problem. He's supposed to take one pill every four hours, not four pills every hour.

The surgical crises' momentum subsided slightly. I settled in with an inexplicably distended abdominal area not unlike the appearance of a third-trimester pregnancy. I was exceptionally uncomfortable, with wild swings from diarrhea to constipation, and on rare occasions I would experience a couple of days reminiscent to what I had previously felt to be normal. Little did I realize that this erratic schedule would become my new normal.

Not Good at Guessing

During the postsurgical visits with my robotic surgeon, we raised repeated questions regarding the abdominal distention. It left us troubled by the nagging concern that it might be signaling a serious problem. On one occasion my wife, who faithfully accompanied me to my appointments, stated that my stomach looked increasingly larger than it had recently. The surgeon assured us that it was fine, while appearing characteristically annoyed by this unexpected delay. Through her persistence, however, he did order a sonogram just to assure her that my abdominal area was in fact normal. To his chagrin, the sonogram revealed that my bladder was dangerously loaded, requiring immediate evacuation.

Consistently Disorganized

I was moved to a room with a patient examination table to permit him to perform a catheterization and relieve the pressure. But an additional problem arose: the staff could not locate an appropriate catheter. It appeared that the office did not have one. Finally, one was discovered, but it proved to be too large. That was acknowledged only after a couple of unsuccessful attempts to insert it. This was extremely painful and all to no avail. I lay on the table, bleeding as a result of these failures. Another smaller catheter was finally located and brought in, and further unsuccessful insertions were attempted. The result was more probing, more pain, more bleeding. Reaching an unbearable pain threshold, I blurted out, "This really hurts like hell." At my indiscretion, he stopped. We were then scheduled for the surgical lab later in the day, and under anesthesia the insertion was successful thus restoring my normal function.

Trust and Verify, or Vice Versa

For decades a culture of camouflage was deemed essential in light of the litigious threats compounded by concealment. It had become a circular threat. The medical and legal professions pointed reproachful fingers while our life-support system of health care suffered amid the conflict. Necessity again becomes the mother of invention. Morbid idioms based on such prickly practices can be diminished by medical transparency. This revolutionary incentive, introduced by increasing numbers of medical professionals to build trust and enhance performance, is a bold new step signaling systemic change. The litigious model based on concealment should begin to recede. "Trust and verify" had, as a response to patients' experience, reversed the polarity to verify and then trust out of necessity—trust in this setting must be earned rather than presumed. A brief reflection of the systemic dysfunction will convince most fair-minded persons that we now need to pursue a common purpose, that of best serving the patient.

A *caveat emptor* posture evolved as a protective mode considered necessary by the patient as a cautious consumer. This became the reality-based admonitory pose derived from the earlier concealment pact that had been adopted as a virtual absolute, albeit unwritten, requirement by medical practitioners. The aphorism about burying mistakes, given that high mortality rate, appeared credible enough to put thinking patients on red alert. A new wave of progressive medical professionals confesses that such a system does in fact exist, is practically universal, and desperately needs revision. The science of medicine will advance by openly acknowledging what worked and what didn't. That will include an accountability assessment from transparent personal performance evaluations. Medical professionals run the gamut, from excellent, good, and fair, to poor and woefully incompetent. Institutions should step forward and accept responsibility for offering patients quality service by policing their profession based on approved standards all can trust. It seems a bit absurd that we have declined the implementation of standards that other vital professions adopted as essential long ago.

A Peek into My Early Surgical Experience

One of my earliest experiences with faulty surgical procedures occurred during my young son's surgery. At the time, I resided in a Northeastern college town for about ten years with my then very youthful family. The community population numbered about four thousand. The historic university was embellished with stylish, collegiate Georgian architecture adorning the brick facade with trendy double-hung windows. It is notable as one of the ten oldest universities in our country. The enrollment was just over eight thousand when we were there and has since doubled. The student body is regarded as conservative and upper middle class. It was accompanied by an adjacent, exclusive women's college of five hundred students, with whom they have merged. The name of the town bespeaks a tribute to historically renowned educational traditions in both the US and abroad.

Surgical Site

While there, our son, about four years of age at the time, developed a hernia on the lower right side of his abdomen that required surgery. The small hospital had three surgeons whose names rhymed, humorously, Drs. Peck, Deck, and Jeck—a neophyte poet's dream for fun and games. The day of my son's scheduled surgery, my wife and I waited anxiously at the small hospital's lounge. After nearly an hour, one of the doctors came charging out. He rather embarrassingly enquired which side the hernia was located on. We informed him that it was on the right side. When my son was lying down, the hernia location was not at all discernible. He looked a bit startled as he hurried back to the operating room.

Surgical Pen Science

The surgery went well, but we noticed a small hint of an incision that had commenced on the left side. That no doubt had occurred before the surgeons abandoned their guessing game and certified the correct site with an appropriate inscription. This was apparently before the medical community had advanced to the science of "error-free procedures," such as distinctly marking "yes" and "no" with a black felt marking pen. That first experience should have been an omen!

Laura Landro in the *Wall Street Journal*[21] filed a report entitled, "Surgeons Make Thousands of Preventable Errors a Year."

---

[21] Laura Landro, "Surgeons Make Thousands of Preventable Errors," *Wall Street Journal*, December 20, 2012.

The study, using data in the National Practitioner Data Bank, a federal repository of medical-malpractice judgments and out-of-court settlements, looked at cases involving leaving an object inside a patient, wrong-site surgeries, wrong procedures and wrong-patient surgeries. . . .

The data extended from 1990 to 2010, and procedures performed on the wrong site were recorded as 24.8 percent of the so-called never events, so labeled given the tragic consequences suffered by the injured patient.

If hospitals were fined $100,000 for a wrong-site surgery, and double that for a repeat incident, "it would make the news, and they would get serious about it," Dr. Leape said.

Our early experience would have been a ringer for the wrong-site fine. Fortunately, the surgeons working on our son had sufficient discernible judgment to ask for directions before blundering ahead and compounding their error of judgment by doing serious harm. My example with my son occurred nearly fifty years ago! They are still doing pretty much the same thing, with little reduction of such tragic errors.

When mistakes are concealed rather than disclosed, practitioners learn very little except for the art of deception.

Dawning Of A New Day In Surgery

I'm so sorry. "Once an X-ray provided proof in black and white, Dr. Das Gupta, the 74-year-old chairman of surgical oncology at the University of Illinois Medical Center at Chicago, did something that normally would make hospital lawyers cringe: he acknowledged his mistake to his patient's face, and told her he was deeply sorry."

The *New York Times*[22] reported Dr. Das Gupta's acknowledgment that "as with any doctor, there had been occasional errors in diagnosis or judgment. But never, he said, had he opened up a patient and removed the wrong sliver of tissue, in this case a segment of the eighth rib instead of the ninth."

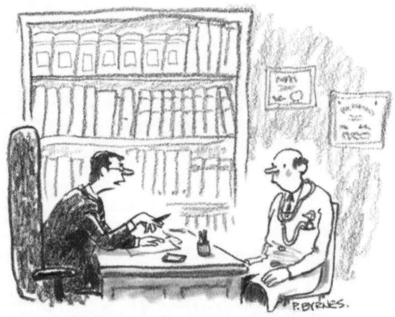

"First, admit no harm."

Dr. Das Gupta confessed to removing a portion of the wrong rib in error. That disclosure to the patient was revolutionary. "After all these years, I cannot give you any excuse whatsoever," Dr. Das Gupta, now seventy-six, said he told the woman and her husband. "It is just one of those things that occurred. I have to some extent harmed you."

---

22   Kevin Sack, "Doctors Start to Say 'I'm Sorry' Long Before 'See You in Court,'" *New York Times*, May 18, 2008.

Trust but Validate

Confusion compounded—I'm sorry too. Shortly after the sudden spate of publications, including this and other related articles, my robotic surgeon suddenly adopted similar verbiage in his routine greeting to me. It was at the time, as you may imagine, an incomprehensible tangled maze of evasion, a statement of apology that in retrospect seems to have been nothing more than a rehearsed parroting of a ritual designed to assure a reduction of enmity. "I am so sorry, so very sorry," lamented my robotic surgeon as he routinely examined my protuberant and conspicuously distended abdomen, which was punctuated with rubber bulbs attached to plastic tubes that protruded from my body to expel collected fluids.

Given the events surrounding my surgery up to that time, this only added to our sense of confusion, concern, and bewilderment. It really served to fuel my suspicions that more serious medical errors had been made, which I suspected from my symptoms but about which I had not been informed. In our local paper, this same surgeon had been dubbed in a headline "Dr. Robot," as the medical community heralded this technologically avant-garde procedure. This was front-page fare shortly before I selected him to remove my cancerous prostate, which enclosed a non–life-threatening malignancy that had not metastasized.

As I abruptly experienced this bizarre, repeated apology on successive visits with no coupled disclosure of medical complications, I found it strange to say the least. In fact, it appeared the converse was implied. My appalling condition was in no way being defined as a consequence of insufficient medical performance on his or anyone else's part. In the context of the aforementioned supportive behavior, I was told repeatedly that I was doing just fine and that my condition was just as it should be—accompanied by the frequently repeated, incomprehensible apology: "I am so sorry." To this day, I remain puzzled by that behavior and even more seriously doubt his integrity as well as his common sense. Was this a strategy he adopted on his own, or was it a collaborative plan shared with others? There was no publically announced design of which I am aware. There appeared to be no such progressive program as those making headlines at that time to undertake a comprehensive reform of their systems.

I developed a totally unremitting distrust of the surgeon's competency and sincerity, and an equally serious concern about his assurances regarding my condition. He was supposed to be the avowed medical expert. Why the abject apology, accompanied by ludicrous, contradictory, and irreconcilable assurances, regarding my circumstances? His peculiar and inconsistent behavior left me in doubt about most anything he said or did, and I also generalized his behavior in part to the medical community there, which he represented.

Medical Malarky

In hindsight, it appears to have been a bizarre and premeditated attempt to piggyback on the publicized benefits of genuine medical reforms initiated and practiced elsewhere. He was misrepresenting my condition while abdicating any responsibility for my hindered progress. By assuming this apologetic posture, detached from reason or disclosure or explanation and not accompanied by any systemic change, it appeared he hoped to harvest the protective benefits (avoidance of legal entanglement) and escape liabilities while assuming a very low esteem regarding my intelligence. His hollow monologues seemed to carry no sincere effort to employ a model of medical integrity. If my assumption is correct, this went well beyond concealment; he was engaging in a more despicable form of deception. I have come to believe that he was keenly aware of incidents that reached the level of significant malpractice inflicted on me (of which I was to remain unaware), and this seemed to be his adopted strategy. An assertive offense is the best defense.

Disclosure of medical errors, followed by sincere apologies and offers of fair compensation for injured patients, were included in the highly innovative and progressive programs that were broadly announced and were genuinely becoming patient-centered. What is now being undertaken is a model designed to enhance standards while attempting to improve medical performance across the board. This would do wonders toward creating a healing atmosphere for patients. The doctor-patient relationships could offer some acceptable basis for restored trust in the medical community.

Chapter Seven

Revenge of the Adhesions

From mid-January 2008 until October, I relished a brief respite where, except for a grossly distended abdomen and bewildering bowel inconsistencies, I returned to a simulacrum of former activity. I deluded myself into thinking that I could enjoy a bit of my prior healthy dietary habits. This was to maintain a high-fiber, low-fat diet with a trace of nuts and fruits, whole-grain bread and cereals, and a glass of red wine with dinner. I have heard the full gamut of expert advice regarding dietary intake for those with compromised colons, from "avoid all fiber" to "it really does not matter." As for the adhesions, they will form in due time, and new complications will be virtually inevitable, independent of dietary selections.

On October 1, 2008, the ominously familiar symptoms of nausea, vomiting, and acute constipation, mysteriously accompanied by chronic hiccups, became the menacing signal for again summoning the ambulance to ferry me to the ER. This routine was distressingly familiar.

"You're Very Unlucky," She Said

My apprehension mounted as I anticipated the unpleasant NG tube thrust into my nostril providing invasive but momentary relief. Nasogastric aspiration though an NG tube is frequently used to remove internal blockages. Looming ahead was the virtually certain life-threatening verdict of surgery as my temporary remedy. The risk of infection, blood loss, anesthesia slip-ups, and all the other agonizingly painful recovery routines flashed across my mind. I was focused enough, however, to be impressed by a sobering, matter-of-fact statement from the attending ER doctor. As she surveyed my distress, she looked me directly in the eyes and announced in an experienced medical tone: "You're very unlucky." What she was sharing with me was the apparent inevitability of recurring problems exacerbated by the merry-go-round of cyclical abdominal surgeries.

Our Paths Will Cross Again

You'll be back, she implied, appearing in no way condescending or intimidating but having summed up my dilemma honestly. As uncomfortable as I was, that honesty was refreshing. What she knew all too well was that abdominal adhesions can be treated, but they are often a recurring problem. Because surgery is both the cause and the cure, the problem can keep returning. For example, when surgery is done to remove an intestinal obstruction caused by adhesions, adhesions may be created by that curative procedure, and form again, bringing new obstructions in at least 10 to 20 percent of patients. In my case it proved to be much higher. The biomechanics of adhesion formation can be readily defined. These abdominal terrorists are at work attacking by stealth. Chemical bonds fasten via tiny collagen fibers as they weave their web of strangulation by embedding in the tissue. The attending ER doctor proved to be prescient in my case. What is intriguing about this encounter is the role she played later in my saga; our paths would cross again in a manner neither of us could really have anticipated at that first meeting.

Notice the references to the adhesion culprits in my medical record, dated October 1, 2008:

Impressions: (1) Small bowel obstruction in the distal ileum in the anterior mid-abdomen. The cause of the obstruction is not seen but likely secondary to adhesions. There is not intra-abdominal abscess, free air, or pneumatosis intestinalis [gas in the bowel wall]. (2) Tethered, matted areas of small bowel are present in the right lower quadrant in the area of the previous abscess. [That abscess location referenced the area of the rectal injury inflicted surgically during the robotic prostatectomy that resulted in the life-threatening hematoma.] (3) Oral contrast has refluxed up the visualized esophagus. The patient should be kept upright or the stomach should be emptied via the NG tube.

Unmentionables: Doctors Are Mum about It

Surgery rescues a portion of the intestines from this insidious strangulation by adhesions—temporarily. That is the deplorable downside in cost and suffering created when anything goes amiss with abdominal surgery. The result, if you survive, is often multiple, repetitive procedures, with diminishing returns as in my case. That surgery is a preview of a seemingly endless series of abdominal invasions, each more risky and insidious than the former. One result of the necessary eviscerations is a decimated, dysfunctional, waning, and totally disfigured midsection as one is left even more vulnerable to further hostile encroachments.

Since this much is understood by the medical community, a penetrating question is in order. Where is the purposeful redress for the patient when the initial surgery is performed ineffectively? Medical professionals fully understand the dire consequences and dangers of the resulting multiple exposures. Should there not be accountability—a sharing of the costs? To ask the question is to answer it. However, it will take invasive transparency to compel accountability, according to disclosing medical professionals. Appropriate incentives will be essential for any established functional systemic change; it will not come by invitation.

How Surgical Errors Stigmatize Patients

Most damaging but seldom clearly portrayed are injuries inflicted by medical practitioners that diminish patients' opportunities for future first-class medical services. A standard of selectivity exists among many quality medical treatment centers. And those of us suffering these injuries are diminished and thereby rendered unqualified for the best care by the limited access. The more compromised the patient's condition becomes from repeated medical errors inflicted by negligent or incompetent treatment, the fewer eminent options remain for that patient. The mathematics of subtraction comes into play. The familiar "three strikes and you're out" is the patient's dilemma too. It carries a comparable onus to that of a preexisting condition. This criterion is often used by hospitals to relegate the patient to a less favorable status for admission, steering them to less qualified professionals—or denying them outright. That recognized deprivation and loss must be factored into the accountability equation. The original medical provider has sabotaged the patient's future prospects. That is doing a lot of harm. Major incentives for improvement in performance and avoiding complications should be invoked. The converse of this would be addressed by responding to incompetent treatment by financially compensating members of the medical community, who would treat the patient and be paid for multiple attempts for a service that should have terminated on the first encounter.

Risk and Mistrust

There was little doubt my attempt to wait out the current dysfunction in hopes of a natural solution was evaporating this time around. The risk I had taken in delaying was driven by my complete mistrust of this medical community—based on my experience from the outcomes of their earlier work. I feared their incompetence from without, more than I feared the blockage threatening from within. What I regard as their ineptitude, based on results, had nearly killed me. I desperately wanted to escape their clutches. I was a captive in their revolving door of cyclic, bungled surgeries, which, as noted above, made them more money via each failure, while taking a further toll on my physical health and endurance.

Experts in the area, as we have seen, readily maintain that each surgery makes the next even more probable and more profitable, depending on the skill of the surgeon, the absence of which (skill, that is) we had encountered all too frequently at the hospital in question. This was coupled with erratic, inconsistent behavior that bordered on the bizarre. I alluded to this earlier in describing my original surgeon. I was very troubled by his contradictory and irreconcilable behavior. Given the concealment pattern, who determines the mental stability and functioning competence of professionals in this closed system? Evidence and probability had taught me to ignore such gestures at my own peril. Remember, you cannot depend on the broken medical system to protect you.

Dr. Gawande, whom I mentioned earlier, tackles this thorny issue, which we appear reluctant to think about. He described an orthopedic surgeon who was the cream of professionals. Wherever he went, it was not long until he was in great demand. He was the doctor's doctor. After a dozen or so years, his workload increased, while his salary more than doubled—and his performance spiraled downward. Routine medical decisions eluded his grasp, and his stellar career came to an abrupt end. That happens more often than we are willing to accept. A significant factor is that doctors are accountable only to themselves, until the botched performances become horrific. In a chapter entitled "When Good Doctors Go Bad,"[23] Gawande writes:

> Doctors are supposed to be tougher, steadier, better able to handle pressure than most. (Don't the rigors of medical training weed out the weak ones?) But the evidence suggests otherwise. Studies show, for example, that alcoholism is no less common among doctors than among other people. Doctors are more likely to become addicted to prescription narcotics and tranquilizers, presumably because we have such easy access to them. Some 32 percent of the general working-age population develops at least one serious mental disorder—such as major depression, mania, panic disorder, psychosis, or addiction—and there is no evidence that such disorders are any less common among doctors. . . . Nonetheless, estimates are that at any given time, 3 to 5 percent of practicing physicians are actually unfit to see patients.

When you come to a fork in the road take it.

—Yogi Berra

Surgery's short shelf life: I desperately needed to try another medical source. What I experienced was akin to surgical Russian roulette. My life was in danger, and I was keenly aware of it. My next surgery would be number three in the same hospital within a single year (between November 2007 and October 2008). A surgical

---

23   Atul Gawande, *Complications: A Surgeon's Notes on an Imperfect Science* (New York: Picador, 2002) p.94

debacle with the initial procedure and a compromised performance with the follow-ups to resolve a deadly hematoma created by the initial surgical failures, all in all, warranted no confidence.

A branch of one of the nation's premier medical providers was located within a hundred miles of my residence. It was close enough to merit a bold and desperate attempt to be my spark of hope. We were also fortunate to have caring relatives residing in that same community who were capable of assisting me.

Trauma by Trauma

Early in the process of waiting out this blockage, Dr. Leader, who appeared to have assumed responsibility for me, came by with a small cadre of interns. This was a part of their routine rounds. Neatly starched white coats formed a ritual horseshoe configuration at my bed with the imposing doctor conspicuously occupying the center. They informed me again of the inherent dangers and the inadvisability of delaying what they described as the inevitable. Both my expectations and the delay, they asserted, were medically dangerous. None dared broach the past surgical procedures and their relationship to the current and additional adhesion formation threatening me, despite the fact that the downside effects of this surgery should be explored openly with patients.

Get Me Out of Here

The discussion soon veered to my concern based on the previous surgeries, which had left me very apprehensive because of the life-threatening complications. To accent my concern, and lacking the basic fundamentals of diplomacy, I opened my hospital gown to unveil a mutilated abdominal area with zigzagging scars, a random patchwork of gross disfigurement, jaggedly etched over my stomach. That gesture and my ill-advised presumptive demeanor ignited the authority figure's combative sensitivity. He instantly took offense. Always in charge, he assumed a confrontational posture. With an air of repudiation and superiority, he informed me that they had in fact saved my life. Based on my medical record, they were involved in both of those problematic surgeries.

I quickly reminded him that I had come to them with a condition that was hardly life threatening—and if he, and they, had indeed saved my life, it was they who had also put it in jeopardy. As we have seen it's a common medical practice: the patient pays for their debacles and pays again as they attempt to rectify them. Such boldness on my part was most unwelcome. I was not conveying the expected obeisance consistent with my assigned subordinate position and social deference. Summing up, I was badly battered but belligerent. I don't recommend it.

Saving the life they had in fact put in peril as spelled out in my medical record hardly afforded them bragging rights, let alone credentialed them for a third experiment at risking my life in order to save it again. In my judgment, my medical emergencies, arising from complications, highlighted their incompetence on that occasion. It was a danger the hospital itself had created. I knew I might not survive the next gamble with them. Recall, they were contacted for assistance to repair the rectal injury during the first surgery. Whatever assistance they may have provided, the outcome of that complication proved devastating.

The future ain't what it used to be.

—Yogi Berra

Here I would like to recount a pertinent earlier experience that involved the rather volatile Dr. Leader. This occurred shortly after my second surgery. As I was slowly recuperating from the hematoma and MRSA infection, my daughter and sons were visiting, and the doctor came by, apparently inspecting the service performance as he passed through. My children mentioned to him that the NG tube was leaking and was in contact with a central line. This, as you may recall, was alluded to earlier as a major source of lethal infections.[24] Dr. Leader immediately called a nurse's attention to that threat. The NG tube had not been properly set to withdraw the fluids and prevent them from collecting in my lungs. Given my condition, this was extremely dangerous, putting me at risk of suffocation and infection. All in the immediate vicinity heard as he spared no feelings in depicting the grave peril to patients that such an oversight could create. Shortly thereafter, I was moved to the trauma level, on another floor, ostensibly to assure closer watch over my care. This appeared to be another example of the failure to properly assign and oversee vital medical services when different departments converged. I was aware of the move but still too medicated to fully appreciate the intended wisdom of this intervention.

I needed another medical source—and I was scrambling. Our spark of hope resided with what we'll call "the Clinic," alluded to above, which was in close proximity, within a hundred miles of my current facility.

---

[24] Landro, p. 9.

The harsh reality was this: In less than a month, as a result of these surgical complications and subsequent infections, I had sustained a hematoma and MRSA infection, followed by months of hospital stays (when taken cumulatively), a thirty-five-pound weight loss, as well as adhesions and other intestinal injuries that were instrumental in these subsequent blocked-bowel surgeries. An otherwise routine surgery had resulted in devastating complications and not an ounce of accountability.

Complications is a code word indicating that things did not go well. Informed patients should acquaint themselves with its significance. How many surgeries a surgeon and an institution have performed is one thing; how many have resulted in complications is quite another. What is their casualty and fatality rate? The answers to these essential, penetrating questions and others could result in your rejection of those hospitals with high negatives. My two very recent surgeries had not gone well at this hospital. Hospitals and doctors do not like to talk about that; but it is information patients need, and the coming systemic change via transparency should help provide it. After this dismal track record, they were asking me to trust them yet again.

Mistrust and Verify

My wife contacted the patient advocacy representative at the hospital and found her most cooperative in attempting to assist us. My wife explained that after two surgeries, with disappointing results, I had no confidence in undertaking a third surgery there. Our request seemed to be reasonable and worthy of her assistance.

I can hardly convey the excitement I felt when informed that I had been accepted at the renowned Clinic. We have a son and daughter who, with their families, live in the city that is in close proximity to the Clinic, and we have a great relationship with them. Travel arrangements were completed, and we were within an hour of departure. With spirits elevated, given my dismal condition, I relished that transfer as would one who had been issued a reprieve from a foreboding sentence. The most dangerous institution in the world was issuing me a reprieve!

Accidental Eavesdropping

My son came by for a morning visit just ahead of our scheduled departure. He boarded the same elevator as the prominent Dr. Leader with whom I'd had the encounter the day before. The doctor was on his cell phone discussing the transfer request of a patient. My son was startled to hear him mention my name to the other party. The person with whom he was conversing represented the safe-haven of the Clinic. Dr. Leader assured this person that any need Mr. Huber had could be met with assurance by Dr. Leader's hospital. The peril involved in a transfer would be an unnecessary risk, he reasoned, and might not be advisable when weighing the dangers involved in travel. What was missing, tragically, from this dialogue was the most important issue, clearly a systemic failure: What are the wishes of the patient? Notice, we had not yet evolved to the level of suitably prioritizing that paramount concern. Upon ending the phone consultation, he then informed the interns that they should make plans to perform the surgery for Mr. Huber!

Experience had recently taught me, painfully, that I did not want a group of medical interns actively participating in my surgery.

Their level of competence was unknown and doubtful at best since experience had not yet refined their potential skills—whatever they might turn out to be—and this was strike three for me. I feared my luck, what little I had in this venture, might soon run out.

It seemed clear to my son from what he had overheard that the doctor's intervention had thwarted all hope of my leaving this hospital for my planned destination of choice. He called me as soon as he exited the elevator and informed me that he had overheard the conversation and the verdict would soon be delivered formally to me. "Dad," he said, "I have disappointing news for you." He then shared the sobering revelation of Dr. Leader's intervention on what I consider his own behalf, not mine. We now had a glimpse of a medical strategy that we would not have been privy to otherwise. My son's chance elevator surveillance and phone interception took me back to square one, and I did not take it well. With all my doubts about their performance up to that point, I naively expected more civil behavior. I was wrong. As I saw it, I had in fact become their hostage.

Chapter Eight

Medical Hostage

Hostage taking is as old as the Bible. There is always a purpose. You don't have to be a tourist in North Korea or venture too close to Somalia to fall prey to a hostage taker. Legislative strategy, too, can be included in this list, as one group will structure clever blocks of voters on issues to force an agenda item not feasible on its own merits. Try the hospital! We would perhaps least expect it there. A fraudulent level is financial, and don't rule that out—they were still making money on me, and they would lose it. Medicine is fundamentally a money business and is really hot for profit, even more so now with Wall Street so heavily involved. Private equity investors, as we shall see, are cleaning up, and we as patients can expect to pay exponentially for any medical screw-ups whenever enhanced profit is the unvarnished purpose of their business.

Another hostage incentive is to prevent the victim from disclosing incriminating information regarding his captors. Put more bluntly, it is the CYA motive: cover your ass. Refusing to acquiesce to your own demise when, from their point of view, burying you would be the least troublesome resolution if you have become their problem is certainly a viable strategy. One certainly shouldn't begin spouting Patrick Henry's "Give me liberty, or give me death." They may be all too willing to accommodate you!

Regardless, as masters, Dr. Leader and his subordinates orchestrated the change in my status. *Master*: just the word here connotes to me the image of total servitude under a lofty superior while pretending you are a patient. I was quite literally the hospital's hostage, and it was for this blink in time my master.

New technology has created a plethora of intriguing designs for controlling subjects. Electronic monitoring is a growing technique. Here, for me, given my physical, financial, and emotional subjugation, and add to that my lack of legal sophistication, I was stuck. I felt as constrained as if I had been thrust into maximum-security solitary confinement. It took a day or so to recover my capacity to think and plan. I had to gather my wits to see if I could survive their captivity with my life. Remember hospitals, by the numbers, are killers—I am not exaggerating the danger. Based on my experience at this institution, and disclosures from medical professionals regarding our jeopardy in hospitals generally, I can say, without doubt, that my life was in grave danger. I am not a paranoid person; in fact, quite the contrary. I'm usually reasonably optimistic. I am also a pragmatist, however; and our reliance must rest, finally, on our reasoning capacity, which is our crowning human achievement.

Having spoken persuasively against my transfer and assuring the prestigious Clinic that his institution was fully capable of providing me with quality care and that I should remain where I was, for my own safety—for the good of the patient—he had grossly misrepresented my circumstances and successfully aborted my transfer, while appearing to be quite reasonable. That was all it took to quash the plan, given the natural disinclination of another hospital to become involved in a medical controversy with a dissatisfied and disgruntled elderly patient, regardless of the circumstances. After all, they might be adversely implicated in future negligence allegations for which they bore no responsibility. Few hospitals wish to risk their reputation on a problem patient, certainly not on one who is not their responsibility and who has been physically harmed.

I believed then, and do now, that the reluctance to facilitate a transfer was predicated in large part on preventing other discerning medical eyes from witnessing my deplorable medically compromised condition, which my current providers had inflicted. They had performed two surgeries, both fraught with serious complications that they desperately wished to conceal. That is the nature of the system. The knowledgeable outsiders would be in a position to raise questions about my condition that could not be subverted by the administrative authority of the hospital or by Dr. Leader's authoritarian presence and influence. An independent assessment or impression appears to have been one of the last things they wished to confront. They had performed terribly, and they knew it. Evidence of harm from the robotic surgery may, given what we now know, have been palpable. His interest seemed to lay more in protecting his hospital than in exhibiting any concern for my welfare. From their vantage point, the damage had been done and had to be concealed— normal medical SOP. The system demanded it. This is despicable, and we must change it.

Within the hour, Dr. Leader and the patient advocate, a thoughtful, petite, and kindly middle-aged lady entered my room to inform me that the Clinic had "changed their mind" regarding my requested transfer. Dr. Leader, always an imposing man, in physical presence as well as demeanor, displayed an authoritarian manner, bordering on the pontifical. He launched in quickly with the air of a victorious conquering adversary inquiring how soon the vanquished patient would choose to acquiesce to an unconditional surrender and undergo the necessary surgery that his hospital so graciously offered.

Having been apprised of the decision prior to his entry, I informed him that I wished to continue with my watch-and-wait strategy until further notice. My trust in that hospital had now plummeted below zero. I knew without doubt I was being kidnapped—held as a patient hostage, against my will—and there was very little I felt I could do to change that. Patient-napping has not made it into our lexicon—yet. I was now in what one might term "medical default," destined to endure another abdominal surgery at the same institution I regarded as responsible for my needing yet another surgery.

Patient-Centered: Someday

Let's pause a moment and contrast this with a hypothetically but unequivocally patient-centered atmosphere. The doctor might have stated clearly that this patient, for whatever reason, had less than complete confidence in his institution. Out of respect for the patient's wishes, he would do all he could to comply with the patient's request and facilitate a successful outcome by assisting with his transfer to the institution of his choice. This accommodating approach is quite incompatible with our current medical culture of concealment. That is the system we have, and it is now being challenged by many in the medical community because they know it harms and kills patients.

So, getting back to reality, I recalled my earlier ER encounter and that doctor's sympathetic assessment of my present condition. Regarding the curse of adhesions, she depicted a discouraging scenario to be played out in my diminishing hope of beating the odds against adhesions and incompetence. She knew all too well the downside of adhesions and was honest enough not to gloss over it. I decided to continue the risk of allowing my body more time to self-correct under the watchful care of the monitoring medical community. It had worked once before when the blockage was in part narcotically induced. I waited and labored for a couple of weeks, roaming the halls, sitting on the commode for a half hour at a stretch—to no avail. Another surgery appeared inevitable, but I still could not mentally override the destructive evidence and manufacture trust in this hospital to perform it.

Many surgeons now prefer laparoscopy as an effective and less invasive procedure for eradicating adhesions. The medical community should consider the importance of sharing with patients its consensus on the most effective procedures, rather than only those their own institution may be adept at using—but profit may be too influential and the patient's benefit too subordinate. In investing, this would be regarded as selling for the house; the brokerage profits first, regardless of the needs of the client. But for long-term health facilitation, that would be a winning strategy for the good of the patient and the health care budget.

Surgeons Impatiently Waiting

Following my ER admission, I was urged and admonished regularly by professionals, apparently eager to have me move into surgery immediately, who brought their touted expertise and the assurance that all would go as well as could be expected. A series of encounters with surgeons, and surgeons to be, had become a significant part of my experience. As I continued my vigil of watchful waiting and hoping, several candidates made their rounds and used the occasion to let me know they were readily available and more than willing. One announced he had recently returned from Iraq, where he had successfully treated the most severely injured, and saved numerous lives. A hint of rewarding medical patriotism accompanied his appeal.

I must assume they felt this to be for my good as well as the facilitation of the hospital's routine schedule of service delivery. Some saw the encounter as an opportunity to caution me of the dangers lurking in my stubborn, if not foolhardy, delay, which could result in intestinal complications that could prove irreparable. My assessment of the real risk to me was too clouded by my unconditional mistrust of this medical community. My previous experience of delaying surgery for a week left me, for better or worse, with the faintest hope that I might recapture that escape from the ravages of another scalpel and another too-early brush with death.

Trust and Vilify

My current pursuit of surgical avoidance proved intensely alienating to the robotic surgeon whom I had seen very infrequently over the past several months. Reports of my watchful-waiting behavior became his growing concern and, I presume, some professional embarrassment. Members of the medical community, whom he now wished to placate, had apparently called my vigil to his attention with urgency and implied responsibility. Perhaps he was genuinely concerned about my welfare independent of how it reflected on him. But his frustration over my behavior proved palpable.

He began an early morning visit with an uncompromising proposition that I discontinue my risky experiment. I reminded him of my inherent mistrust because of inferior outcomes and the deliberate sabotaging of my efforts to transfer to the Clinic. He adopted the party line, suggesting that it was most likely that the Clinic wished not to become involved with a disgruntled patient reacting negatively to the current supportive medical community. Patients are most often wrong in their medical judgment, he asserted. Even if the patient's position is credible, he has no rights that will merit reflection in this highly esteemed medical court of no confidence.

This Patient Is Not a Robot

Though the robotic doctor's view may have represented traditional medical decision making, within the system, my own reaction was to emphasize the inherent lack of fairness in this process. It is morally wrong to condemn the patient to treatment by those in whom he has justifiably lost all confidence. It was apparent that my concept of fairness was an unwelcome intruder in this medical arena; and from what I could see, it was the last thing being considered.

Rant and Rave

His temper tantrum came as a complete surprise; it stood in a class by itself. Most of his consultations were likely with patients who routinely did what they were told by the medical community, and especially by their surgeon. The conundrum here was that this patient had lost complete confidence in those who were now attempting to enlist his cooperation, ostensibly for his own good. The superior medical authority derived from their touted expertise no longer carried persuasive influence since I no longer trusted them. They had ceased to represent my best interests; now their own interests, and not my wellbeing, were at stake.

In this latest conversation with the robotic surgeon, I was not persuaded but continued my resistance. He suddenly became enraged and lectured me heatedly in ominous tones. He began in decipherable English and then veered into a dialect I failed to recognize. His intensity was so hyperactive I became fearful that he was going to attack me physically. His face was flushed as he swiftly pivoted and left my room. I thought that was the last I might ever see of him—and with that thought, I was momentarily relieved.

Never Saw Him Again

In a few minutes he returned. His civil demeanor restored, he told me that I needed to seriously consider his and his colleagues' wishes for me to behave in my own best interest and get on with the recommended surgery. He then departed, and this was in fact the last time I saw him.

I was convinced that most of my current difficulties originated from the first robotic surgical procedure. I wished to enlist the best surgeon available to perform the looming third surgery—my life depended on it.

Chapter Nine

Challenging the Medical Status Quo

Fully cognizant that this was a teaching hospital, I wanted to avoid being sacrificed as a practice dummy for inexperienced students in training. The previous surgeries had been the extent of my contribution in that regard. Lay wisdom urges the vetting of a surgeon since, as some medical experts are now acknowledging, some are incompetent. This vetting process should include questions regarding the number of previous identical surgeries he or she has performed. If that number is below two hundred—look elsewhere. Include in that request, the question of how many resulted in complications. Interns will seldom have the bare minimum experience, or may even have none at all. In fact your surgery may be their very first. After all, they must start somewhere..It might as well be at your risk, even if it means your life. It is for a good cause!

As we have seen earlier, doctors themselves are much less generous in permitting interns and residents to have access to them or members of their own families, based on their actual experience. When that segregation of practice for patients only is rectified, we will have significantly improved medical professionals. If the interns are not good enough for the doctors' families, they are not ready for mine; I care about both.

Their educational experience, as presently conducted, can be quite costly to patients. In most cases that practice on you and me is done surreptitiously. It is an issue of contention among medical educators as to whether patients should be informed at all, as though it might be none of our business. If that is the case, there is something seriously dubious about this facet of the medical business. The point I wish to make here is that we should be consulted in advance and given the right of refusal (with no negative consequences). Many doctors are convinced that patients should not be asked or informed. That is another medical practice that you may well find offensive, and you should. Patients are put at risk here, and as we have seen, the negative consequences can be devastating and irreversible.

I recall a crude attempt at humor depicting the patient having been prepped and wheeled on the gurney toward the operating room: "Doctor, this is my first operation, and I am terribly nervous," says the patient. "You can relax," the comforting doctor responds. "This is my first surgery too!"

On the other side of surgery, that ceases to be as funny

Since I was in essence being forced to undergo the procedure there, my dilemma was how to be assured that I had the best doctors possible. I, as a patient, wished to have a choice in that selection. In my experience, past performance was incredibly relevant. But what alternatives did a medical hostage have?

Kidnapper to the Rescue!

Double-edged scalpel: Dr. Leader, described earlier in that confrontational bedside scene, had a respectable reputation for abdominal surgery, as I had come to learn. I investigated as carefully as possible, given my circumstances. He kept emerging as a serious candidate—and for reasons in addition to his reputed surgical skills;

the fledgling interns and residents would not mess around with this kidnapper!

Among the critical variables, in addition to his reputed surgical skill, were the need for a controlling influence over the interns, which was often lacking. Horror stories abound regarding the tragic results of their rudimentary attempts at surgery. Many have been known to feign experience they don't have in order to get a leg up on their peers. "Competition is fierce!" they protest. "You gotta do what you gotta do." I had too much at stake here to tolerate those with "fake it 'til you make it" training credentials.

How Not to Become a Buried Mistake

I drew some reassurance from the knowledge that this doctor, if he accepted responsibility for the outcome, given his temperament, was known to strike fear into the most stalwart medical students and even other professionals on his watch. This helped to increase my assurance of a survivable outcome. Anyone assisting, whose performance would reflect on him, had better not screw it up! Heads could roll if he were made to appear to be less than the best. It was a calculated decision, given the limited options available to me from my dungeon of captivity. He appeared to be my best bet. It was a gamble, but I was willing to take it if he would consent—so he did, and I did. And I am still alive to write this!

The potential calamity for the patient is obvious here, as I have stated. When the patient's medical treatment results in serious complications, the system thrusts the resulting pain, suffering, and financial sacrifice squarely onto the back of that patient. If they survive they are financially strapped, incurring all the expense of complications, repeated procedures needed, and other injuries and losses sustained. A big "if" since they have an earned reputation for burying their mistakes with impunity. The medical professionals continue to be fully compensated for appalling performances. Accountability is not yet a trustworthy issue—no consistent incentive here for quality, no need to learn from their mistakes. This is a real "moral hazard" (to borrow a euphemism from Wall Street) with their ineluctable history.

Poop to the Rescue?

Eureka! A couple of days prior to the scheduled surgery, the toilet vigil appeared to offer a hint of success. I never thought I would be so excited over a little poop! I summoned the nurse in triumph. She verified the contents and hastily called an intern on duty. The intern's response was intimidating, with an interrogating, "How can we be sure that it's yours?" Was I giving her the straight scoop on my poop? After a moment of perplexed speculation, I muttered a silly, "DNA would prove it." After that insipid challenge, I was too pooped to continue. I had given them the honest-to-poop truth. So in the presence of the two ladies staring at my brown droppings, I only managed to flush a blush and head to bed. Upon reflection I have to consider that I had voiced a less-than-favorable opinion of the competency level of the interns, of which they were well aware. Thus the intern's attitude toward me, on this occasion, is not surprising. This is an important thing for patients to remember.

As I was informed elsewhere later on by more patient-centered professionals, a colonoscopy may well have been a preferred treatment in such circumstances and an invasive and destructive surgery prevented or delayed for a substantial period of time. I was given no such consideration or instruction, nor was this even discussed for that matter. Surgery was job one! With the emphasis on hospital management by profit, driven by private equity investors, more money likely would be gained by surgery anyway. Profit in medicine is often an end in itself—keep that in mind. Surgery had been planned, and the appearance of poop was a vile and offensive intrusion. Another option was not offered me, and I was too unsettled to press for further consideration.

Revolving Door

As you will note from the operative report quoted more extensively below:

"Mr. Huber is a pleasant gentleman WELL KNOWN [*caps mine*] to our service for small-bowel obstruction." An ill-omened compliment exceptionally predictive of future crises. He should at least have added, "We certainly played a significant role in his being here today—adhesions generating, hostage taking, etc." Since the repetitive scenario was initiated by the role they had played, it again raises the specter of concealment versus transparency and accountability. There was never the hint of their accepting any responsibility for their involvement in the permanently diminished quality of my life resulting from these medical complications. Only irrefutable transparency will usher in accountability. As we have noted recently, rebellion is rising in the ranks. As a patient living with the aftermath of these poorly performed abdominal invasions, I was caught in a revolving door. Abdominal surgery, adhesions, obstruction, abdominal surgery, adhesions, obstruction, surgery, ad infinitum. The predicted systemic changes regarding opacity versus transparency and the measured acceptance of responsibility would be most welcome.

"You're Very Unlucky" Returns

Our patient-centered ER doctor (of the "you're very unlucky" candor), who had acknowledged the perils of repeated abdominal surgeries, entered our lives again. She turned out to be the famed Dr. Leader's surgical assistant of choice for my operation. She had educated me on postsurgical bowel obstructions via adhesions, which appeared to be the repetitive culprit, resulting in small intestine blockages a high percentage of the time.

She came by my room the day prior to my scheduled operation, as my son was visiting, reiterated the formal cautionary information, and obtained the signatures required prior to all surgeries. These releases of responsibility cover the broad state statutory limit of liability, which must be agreed to as an entry requirement for admission to the hospital and surgery. They are restrictive to the degree that they put the patient in a virtual legal chokehold, substantially reducing the hospital's financial liability—and that purposely calibrated and insignificant sum would hardly begin to fund a serious legal challenge for careless medical procedures, making litigation in that arena very difficult and less likely. The ER doctor appeared genuinely sympathetic about my multiple complications and recounted her own experience with a close relative who had faced equally trying medical outcomes with life-altering consequences.

Chapter Ten

Third Surgery

Just prior to the surgery as I waited to be taken to the OR, I requested a brief audience with my surgeon captor. I was informed that he had already scrubbed and prepared for the procedure, so a visit would be very inconvenient. But I insisted, wisely or unwisely. I wanted to make sure he was actually there and committed to his promise to complete the surgery himself. Within five minutes, both he and our "you're very unlucky" doctor appeared at the curtain, attired in their surgical dress. They were very pleasant and assured me that all would be carried out just as we had agreed.

Postoperative Diagnosis: Small-bowel obstruction, malnutrition, internal hernia with volvulus times two . . .

Indications for Procedure: Briefly, Mr. George Huber is a pleasant gentleman well known to our service for small-bowel obstruction. He failed medical management and ultimately presented to the Operating Room for surgical intervention. . . . Incision was made along the midline from the sternum to pubis along the previous scar. . . . The small bowel was immediately noted to be quite distended. . . . Two internal hernias with volvulus were identified. The first one was identified at the level of the mid to distal jejunum. The second was identified at the terminal ileum. Both of these internal hernias were reduced. The bands (adhesions) causing the internal hernia were lysed and all bowel was viable. . . . All adhesions were lysed. . . . It was determined the patient would benefit from placement of a nasojejunal tube, for his malnutrition. . . . The nasojejunal tube was secured with tape.

In order to facilitate placement of the bowel back into the abdominal cavity the nasojejunum tube was placed on suction and the obstruction fluid was milked proximally and distally. The bowel was easily returned to the abdominal cavity. The subcutaneous tissue was irrigated with normal saline. The skin was closed with staples.

Dr. Leader, following the surgery called my wife and informed her that the operation had gone well and an intern was closing the incision. I developed a suture complication that lasted several months after the surgery. The record indicates staples were used for the closure. That is consistent with our recollection, as I was examined following the staple removal and dismissed to the care of my GP. Several weeks after the surgery, I began experiencing redness and irritation just below the belt line. The site also became infected a couple of times. The cause appeared to be a troublesome suture. We had been informed that any remaining sutures would dissolve. My GP, after a considerable time, having made several unsuccessful attempts to remove it, referred me to the hospital. He was trying to help me, since I was very reluctant to return to the hospital that had taken me as a medical hostage. I had taken a couple of doses of antibiotics for my concern about a MRSA infection; and fearing further complications, I consented to return to the hospital for assistance as an outpatient.

An intern attempted to remove the object without success. He then called his senior intern, who promptly came in, with bare hands, and found the task more complicated than he expected. He then assembled several instruments and began in earnest. After a bit of a struggle, he was able to remove it. Out of curiosity, I asked him to give it to me, wanting to show it to my GP, but the senior intern informed me that he had to discarded it as medical waste. It was black and very stiff, more than an inch long, with the appearance of a piece of thin coat hanger wire. I expressed concern regarding why it had been put in my stomach and who had decided to do so, but I received no additional information from the intern.

It would not have dissolved. I assume whomever Dr. Leader had delegated to suture the incision must have put it there. It caused me six months of discomfort and concern, as well as two doses of antibiotics to stave off infection because of the sensitive location and our concern about MRSA.

I share this because you can't be sure who will be working on you in the seclusion of the OR—and what level of experience or inexperience they will have. This is yet more evidence of the need for transparency.

My medical record regarding this procedure stated, "The subcutaneous tissue was irrigated with normal saline. The skin was closed with staples." As a patient I would assume the hospital and physician in charge would be very concerned about such irregularities—they seemed not to be.

Stop Taking Your Damn Temperature!

Infection is the number-one killer following surgery. It is heralded by the presence of persistent fever. I developed a low-grade fluctuating fever prior to my dismissal from the hospital following surgery. I was especially hypersensitive about it since this was the cautionary symptom—an apprehensive prelude to a serious, even fatal, abdominal infection.

As we were nearing the target date on the dismissal schedule, I shared this ongoing concern with my surgeon—bad timing! I had raised the issue of my temperature again since it was not yet down to normal without forcing it medically. He was dismissive in his memorable and inimitable style: "Stop taking your damn temperature!"

I assume that I caught Dr. Leader when he had more important things to be concerned about. He had weighty administrative responsibilities. I remember thinking again, *This is an unsafe, insalubrious place!* I must reiterate—and I seriously believe—that our medical professionals are functioning in a system that is tragically flawed. They are not villains, and most of us, were we to trade places, would behave comparably. We must change the system.

His manner, body language, and scowling facial expression all bespoke his disdain and derision for me, his patient. Here he made no attempt to conceal his disrespect. I was, to him, that outsider, unworthy of his medically consistent attention or respect. I seemed to be an inconsequential distraction from what he regarded as his mission; his purpose, whatever it was, certainly was not me. Even with this eruption, I felt gratitude—he had gotten me out the door alive!

Following this additional rotation in my adhesion's relentless revolving door, I was released from my captivity, the hospital, on Thursday, October 23, 2008. With that third surgery completed, again I felt so lucky to be alive because I was now acutely aware of the danger. That was a lengthy hospital experience with which I should have been accustomed by this time; but it remained an abhorrent challenge. Captivity on that occasion, as always, had included sleep deprivation due to scheduled and unscheduled interruptions, room sharing when private accommodations were unavailable, and constant people traffic and noise, to cite a few reasons. And on top of it all, as I had come to understand, this was by far the most dangerous, the deadliest, institution.

Temp Up—Back to Er

Following my release and brief convalescence, progress was interrupted by another alarming fever. My previous experience with a hematoma had left me apprehensive, especially since it had been exacerbated by MRSA. For those not familiar with this term, methicillin-resistant *Staphylococcus aureus* (MRSA), is a bacterium that has been responsible for many serious infections. The bacterium is highly resistant to modern drug treatment and as a result can be deadly. A fever could easily represent a new MRSA progression.

My temperature kept slowly creeping up, and my instructions were to call medics daily. Given such symptoms, this could be serious. When a fever of 102 F lingered for the better part of a day, I went to the ER to determine the cause. The ER was my only way to reenter the hospital. The pleasant but overworked staff in the ER were trying hard to serve, but for patients it required insufferable waiting. Three hours crept by. About 2:00 a.m., while attempting to get to the bathroom, I passed out. Good fortune placed me by a very alert gentleman who was accompanying a relative and, witnessing my collapse, intercepted my fall.

That episode attracted the attention of a staff member who feared a heart attack and quickly hurried me into a wheelchair. I was hustled to the examination room. Thankfully, it was not my heart. However, my blood profile indicated I needed a transfusion, badly. Two units were administered as soon as they could clear me.

Replacing Blood Loss

Ideally, blood loss should be replaced with crystalloid or colloid solutions to maintain intravascular volume (normovolemia) until the danger of anemia outweighs the risks of transfusion. At that point, further blood loss is replaced with transfusions of red blood cells to maintain hemoglobin concentration (or hematocrit) at that level. For most patients, that point corresponds to a hemoglobin between 7 and 10 g/dL (or a hematocrit of 21–30%). Below a hemoglobin concentration of 7 g/dL, the resting cardiac output has to increase greatly to maintain normal oxygen delivery.[25]

Tests also indicated that I was low on potassium (a condition called hypokalemia; potassium is critical for nerves and muscles including the heart muscles), which is very dangerous for anyone, especially the elderly. The attending nurse seemed confused and perplexed when saddled with the responsibility of resurrecting me from this brush with another medical disaster. I required an intravenous application, which had to be calibrated precisely to be administered safely. I was scheduled to be dismissed that day (they needed the room). It appears there was more incentive for them in my leaving than in my remaining in the hospital. This was the same hospital that had patient-napped me the previous month . Now they were quite eager to get rid of me.

Coming to Our Senses

Remember, I was still under the supervision of the prominent Dr. Leader, who had been instrumental in taking and holding me

---

[25] G. Edward Morgan Jr. and Maged S. Mikhail, *Clinical Anesthesiology* (New York: Appleton and Lange, 1996). See also: http://www.manuelsweb.com/ blood_loss.htm and http://www.ncbi.nlm.nih.gov/pmc/articles/PMC2918661/

hostage less than a month before and who was now pressed by different incentives. This was the same man who had gone into a bit of a conniption regarding my concern about my elevated body temperature. Again this could be confirming evidence for why medical professionals have begun sounding their own alarms concerning the dangers for patients. The system in which they must function is not patient-centered.

I noticed my indecisive nurse was irresolute about the proper formula for the administration of the potassium dosage. She appeared to have nowhere to turn. It was now Saturday afternoon, and Monday was a holiday, Veteran's Day. My hospital doctor might have been ticked off at the very mention of my temperature; and my nurse was unnerved about the dosage of potassium. This was not a safe place— double jeopardy. One did not know, and the other seemed too busy to be bothered. Stress is not healthy. I decided to meditate right there on the spot.

Meditation for a Medicated Mind

I had a little experience with progressive relaxation and self-hypnosis but no formal or certified training. Somebody in that room needed to be relaxed—might as well be me. I tried to recall my ritual starting with my toes and moving slowly to the top of my head. Little by little the script reappeared in my mind. Here is a brief sample in case you should ever find such rituals helpful. I vocalized silently in my mind:

> I am beginning to relax, breathing naturally, very slowly now, paying attention to the bottom of my feet, moving slowly upward until my toes and the tops of my feet are in my awareness. Next my ankles . . . my calves . . . my knees . . . my thighs, moving so slowly.

Medical Madness

Next my buttocks, abdomen, my waist are in my awareness. Next my hands, my forearms, upper arms, my chest, shoulders, neck, chin, jaws, my mouth, nose, eyes, and forehead. Very slowly, going up over my scalp and the top of my head, my whole body is relaxed, very, very relaxed, breathing naturally.

Feel myself drifting slowly downward now, slowly, very deep, very deep, very, very deep. Very far down. I am healthy, very, very healthy, from the top of my head to the bottom of my feet. My emotions and outlook are positive. Every event I regard positively. I am very relaxed. I am drifting downward slowly, very slowly and very deep. I am now confident, competent, and compassionate. I believe in compassion and optimism to direct everything that I do. Drifting slowly into the deepest relaxation.

This took about fifteen minutes.[26]

There were several occasions in which I practiced a mindfulness ritual that I had acquired through my reading, and I made a habit of doing it several times a week. *Time* magazine carried a cover story on mindful meditation quite recently that followed the experiences of people who received formal training in the practice. One point is worth noting:

> A related and potentially more powerful factor in winning over skeptics is what science is learning about our brains' ability to adapt and rewire. This phenomenon, known as neuroplasticity, suggests there are concrete and provable benefits to exercising the brain. The science—particularly as it applies to mindfulness—is far from conclusive. But it is another reason it's difficult to dismiss mindfulness as fleeting or contrived.[27]

---

[26]   Jon Kabat-Zinn, *Coming to Our Senses: Healing Ourselves and the World Through Mindfulness, Lying Down Meditations* (New York: Hyperion, 2005).

[27]   Kate Pickert, "The Art of Being Mindful," *Time*, February 3, Vol. 183, NO 4, 2014, p.43. Time & Life Building, Rockefeller Center, New York, New York. 100200-1393

In the hospital you should always use all the help you can get. Sometimes when things seem normal, a surprise lurks nearby.

An additional issue appeared, impeding my departure: my potassium level was still too low. The nurse had been indecisive in grasping the proper intravenous application of potassium; she made an attempt but was not familiar enough with the procedure to get the potassium level near normal.

Late Saturday afternoon, November 8, 2008, with my potassium still low but assuming I had received enough to stay alive for a couple of days, the medical professionals checked me out, with orders to contact my general practitioner as soon as possible. Monday was a holiday, so I could not get an appointment until 4:15 p.m. to complete the potassium dosage. Since the potassium was still quite low, we got a prescription to elevate it: orange-flavored potassium bicarbonate effervescent tablets oral solution, 25 mEq (977 mg). I was to take it three times a day. I dropped a tablet into 4 ounces of cold water and watched as it created a fascinating, fizzed-up little spectacle. My GP of several years called later that same evening to make sure everything was OK. I breathed a sigh of relief. I was alive and out of the hospital. It is most always safer on the other side—while still alive! Additional sutures and staples from surgery were removed on November 18, 2008, and I was placed on routine follow-up.

Chapter Eleven

Red Alert

A scheduled visit to my hematologist a month later resulted in an immediate hospitalization for three additional units of blood. I was sent directly from his office to the hospital. The surgical procedure for abdominal obstructions on October 17, 2008 may have generated substantially more blood loss than was reported at the time. The record indicates that the estimate of blood loss was 80 mL. I experienced excessive fatigue in the weeks following the surgery, and my collapse in the emergency room was consistent with the hematologist's findings. On that occasion they had issued two units of blood, which was insufficient.

If you don't know where you are going, you
might wind up someplace else.

—Yogi Berra

Scrap That MRI

While hospitalized this time, I underwent several tests to determine the cause of my chronic anemia; this had been diagnosed originally several years earlier but was apparently stabilized for the time being. I had undergone a bone marrow biopsy in 2006, which was negative. Now the medical team attending me requested an MRI of my abdominal area to look more closely at my liver. The test was completed, but evaluation of the results was promptly cancelled without my being consulted. Another team member ordered a biopsy of my liver instead. I went from the MRI (completed but not evaluated) in the early afternoon to a liver biopsy by midafternoon.

Bring on the Biopsy

The medical team seemed undecided about which tests and procedures to require. There appeared to be no apparent comprehensive plan or regular communication within the group regarding what was to be accomplished and how to proceed. The lack of effective organization, here of all places, should not be the norm—life and death are in the balance. A reminder: this is a consistent criticism of the medical community now being leveled repeatedly by professionals from within. Situations can and often do end tragically; patients are irreparably harmed, and many die because these issues leave room for serious errors. Take it from an injured patient with complications, when lives are at stake, get it right the first time! Team communication in the medical environment should be excellent because of the very nature of their work. Instead, it is frequently nonexistent.

Lights On and Keep 'Em On!

The liver biopsy fared little better than the MRI. It was accented by a game of "Who needs the lights?" A pleasant and personable nurse prepped me and gave me a local anesthesia with 1 percent buffered lidocaine. The supporting staff appeared somewhat puzzled with the lighting source. As the physician readied the probe under ultrasound guidance, the lights went out. A slight commotion followed. I then heard a commanding male voice: "I need the lights!" The lights went on in a different area, and shortly thereafter, we had our lights again. Then in the middle of another probe, the lights disappeared again. A bit more irritated, the physician called out, "The lights, please!" Then on a subsequent probe the lights blinked again, momentarily, and finally the assistants grasped and mastered their seemingly complex light-switch maze. That event, after the MRI caper, was not at all reassuring.

Flickering Lights and a Faulty Test

Perhaps this is understandable since it was a few days prior to Christmas (mustn't expect too much). A total of three passes were made to harvest the necessary samples. The results, however, failed to present evidence of a liver abnormality that would explain the chronic anemia—so another test for a liver biopsy was ordered without consulting me or explaining the need for it.

I soon learned the defective report had been returned, as flawed as our lights-capade. It appeared an essential component had not been requested. Apparently the liver culture sample had not been placed under observation for the required seventy-two hours to determine if it had undergone an observable change. That rendered the test defective. I received a call informing me that an appointment for a CT scan had been ordered to determine if the liver sample, when contrasted with the one taken prior to the first biopsy, revealed sufficient change to warrant a repeated biopsy.

Do It Over Again

The CT scan as interpreted, provided adequate variation so the doctors could proceed with the second biopsy. (I wonder if such evidence would have been palpable if not for the prior decision to rectify a faulty first procedure. I have no hard evidence of this; it's just a hunch.) The anticipated risk, exposure, and discomfort annoyed me to the point that I was quite unpleasant with the assistant (who was, after all, only acting as the messenger), and I felt badly afterward. She was just doing her job. I indicated that the biopsy had been very painful and might be unnecessarily invasive for one my age. The CT scan exposes one to radiation equivalent to a thousand X-rays. It seemed the specialist and I were avoiding confrontation with each other, and the assistant was caught between us. I still regret that, yet lament even more the bungling medical treatment that has endangered my life since the first surgical debacle. These repeated foul-ups are a stark reminder of the dangers we all face.

The same physician who had completed the previous liver biopsy performed the second as well. He was apologetic to me and insisted that he had conducted the first test precisely as requested, flickering lights notwithstanding. The implication was that someone had erred, but it was not his fault. This still lives vividly in my memory since on the second biopsy, my blood pressure dropped well below normal and I had to remain under observation for substantially longer than routinely expected.

A member of the team, assessing my condition on the original hospital visit (where we had endured the blinking-lights episode), commented regarding the earlier liver test that after three surgeries, with liver available and under surveillance, sufficient opportunity existed to ascertain those abnormalities. He was a member of the team and obviously skeptical. However, I was relieved when, in the final analysis, the seventy-two-hour petri dish culture did not reveal any observable activity.

In summary, I had a completed and then discarded MRI, an inadequately performed liver biopsy, and an additional CT scan (with very high radiation exposure) to validate a repeat biopsy. The three units of blood I desperately needed to bring me up from the recent surgery were very helpful. And of course, these risks and costs had all been borne in the final analysis by me, the patient. This was sloppy medicine and unworthy of the highly credentialed leaders engaged. Was anyone in charge? Again, this underscores a fundamental criticism leveled at the medical community, charging them with a lack of organization and teamwork that repeatedly endangers the lives of their patients. The system strikes again.

My affirmation of respect and gratitude for my hematologist is overdue here. He has been trustworthy and available and has intervened effectively in my crucial and perilous surgical experiences in ways that have allowed me to be present now to pursue this narrative. Given the dangers of surgery and my consistent problem with blood loss, it is very reassuring to have a dedicated, knowledgeable, and caring professional assisting and helping bring about a favorable outcome. I am continually grateful.

Chapter Twelve

How Surgeries Kill

Surgery is a very dangerous procedure. Dr. Atul Gawande has documented consistent variables worldwide and attempted to reduce the mortality rates by describing what has been learned collectively over time. Thanks to this information, thousands of lives have been saved, including mine and perhaps yours as well.

> Surgery has, essentially four big killers wherever it is done in the world: infection, bleeding, unsafe anesthesia, and what can only be called the unexpected. Research conducted by the World Health Organization, WHO, found that guidelines regarding these variables reduce complications and mortality rates dramatically.[28]

Medical Marathon

This account is offered to assist readers' understanding of my experience. The first medical procedure on November 19, 2007, stretched into a marathon. As numerous complications mounted, natural or negligent, they threatened an orderly process and my life. In less than a month, as a result of the previously described developments, I found myself on the road to numerous medical procedures. The resulting medical events—subsequent infections, a hematoma, MRSA, a couple of months of cumulative hospital stays, drastic weight loss of twenty-five percent, numerous adhesions and

---

[28] Gawande, Atul *The Checklist Manifesto: How To Get Things Right*. (New York: Picador, 2010). P. 101

other intestinal disruptions,—required subsequent blocked-bowel surgeries. This errant first surgery and the bungled attempts to correct the damage appear to be the primary cause of what followed.

Keep in mind this originated from an otherwise routine surgery with avant-garde technology and devastating consequences for which I alone bore the cost and suffering, with no institutional accountability or compensation. The hospital has never acknowledged responsibility, consistent with our medical system of concealment.

Routine Patient Punishment

My wife and I were deprived personally and financially, while the medical community has not been held accountable, required to admit errors or offer any corrective compensation. There are currently lawsuits against the robotic surgery manufacturer and various surgeons. But the problem goes deeper than individual episodes.

The current system in place fails to encourage the rehearsal of medical procedures to determine what might be done to assure a more positive outcome in subsequent surgeries. That review, essential for medical progress, is regarded as too revealing, it's an admission of error. Bad incentives are systemic, concealment is more important than improvement in a science on which all our lives depend. Fairness to patients and advancement in medical practice should be paramount; the system is in dire need of improvement. I pose this question to the medical authorities: how would you proceed if you or members of your family were the patients in cases like mine? Now get busy doing it.

Eight-Hundred-Pound Gorilla

The dominating medical service delivery system in the area—in terms of size, history, variety and complexity of services provided—could not prevent the influence and power it wields even if it tried. Such dominance is a double-edged sword. How professionals respond to this authority varies considerably.

Clinical Prognosis: Distended Colon, Surgery Suggested

Some medical representatives were sympathetic to my discomfort but appeared inaudibly reluctant to pursue analyses that might clash with certain previous, inferior medical procedures responsible for my condition. This concerned me because it gave the impression that this tension affected what they were doing to help me. It seemed tacitly understood but always unspoken. In the meantime, I had monitored with daily apprehension the abdominal distention that was possibly evidence of a pending medical crisis. I wanted to prevent another sudden abdominal surgery.

Code of Silence Invoked

The apparent disinclination to be open and candid is understandable. It was systemically conforming but morally indefensible. I came to regard this culture of concealment as a medical hindrance even to my treatment regimen. Betraying the cardinal premise of that unwritten code could have serious career implications. It is easy to understand the impact of the power of concealment in the medical community, enforced from the top down via an understood commitment. That game must be played at all levels to be most effective. Generally, doctors seldom venture a denigrating assessment of other doctors regardless of whether poor results stem from deviant behavior or are the consequences of an inferior performance.

"See no evil" descends from the highest echelons of the medical organization to the lowest rungs on the ladder. Referrals, the lifeblood of a robust profession, may dwindle and cease if betrayal is detected. It remains fully understood that loyalty is obligatory. In my own case, this concept was awkwardly controversial inasmuch as it involved the most influential medical institution in the area, responsible for my past surgeries and complications. Careers flourish or flounder based on adherence to the code of silence; yet this was doing substantial harm to the patient and retarded progress in the medical community. Failures can be instructive, if faced; they are overcome, and then seldom repeated. That requires accepting accountability.

Patients are permanently harmed within this culture. This raises the specter of concealment and disloyalty to the patient, a real double whammy. An often-overlooked complication is that inferior status is attributed to the one who has become medically injured. Even the best institutions commonly practice this discrimination. The patients are then relegated in status to shunned patients. They become virtually untouchable because of their compromised health and its accompanying negative risk to the highly esteemed institutions. If these institutions embrace a seriously injured and permanently compromised patient as a result of complications, their qualitative outcomes are diminished. Successful treatment outcomes for an previously injured patient are difficult to evaluate precisely.

As damaged patients, we are drastically restricted and prevented from getting the best treatment available in the future as a direct result of the medical harm inflicted on us. One has now acquired the stigma equivalent to a preexisting medical condition. The penalty for being put into this situation is medical abandonment—you are barred from access to the highest-quality treatment. Our chances of rehabilitation are reduced, inasmuch as the preferred medical treatment is now out of reach. It is a crude comparison, but it's similar to the loss in value of a vehicle that has incurred damage due to being involved in a serious accident.

The *Wall Street Journal* describes attempts by Dr. Marty Makary to bring transparency and accountability to the medical profession:

> In "Unaccountable," Marty Makary offers a searing indictment from the inside, arguing that the modern health-care industry, unlike almost every other, doesn't disclose its performance or pricing practices to the public and keeps under wraps information about mistakes and substandard quality.
>
> As a surgeon at Johns Hopkins Medicine in Baltimore and a professor of health policy at Johns Hopkins's Bloomberg School of Health, Dr. Makary isn't just a disgruntled whistleblower. He has seen much of what he writes about—and readily confesses his own complicity over the years in concealing the flaws of medical care from those who stand to lose the most when it goes wrong: patients.
>
> In the course of his long career he has encountered all manner of malfeasance. He describes a surgeon who removed half a patient's colon through a large abdominal incision to take out a polyp that could have been removed simply with a wire snare—except the surgeon wanted to do it his way rather than call in a colleague with expertise in the less invasive procedure.[29]

---

[29]   Laura Landro, "Hospital Horrors: Meet 'Shrek,' a Doctor Who Insists on Surgery in Every Case—and Has a Surgical-Incision Infection Rate of 20%," *Wall Street Journal*, October 3, 2012.

Acceptance: Too Little, Too Late

I had applied to the renowned Clinic, but as described earlier, the dominant Dr. Leader thwarted my efforts through his phone intervention. Considerably later, after several attempts, the Clinic approved my application to enter for a complete physical. I was concerned primarily with the repeated intestinal blockages but felt I might have a better chance if I entered on the premise of a complete physical workup. I had three days of extensive testing, the most complete physical I have ever experienced. As I feared, they found a developing blockage, an imminent and life-threatening intrusion. I quote my record from their institution:

> GI evaluation. Anorectal function test revealed a pelvic floor dysfunction. CT enterography revealed findings consistent with intermittent sigmoid volvulus. The stomach was dilated there was soft tissue thickening [adhesions again!] of the antrum. . . . Dr. Smith recommended referral to [the Clinic's] Colorectal Surgery for evaluation.

Therein Lie the Ghosts from Surgeries Past

Evidence shows that multiple abdominal surgical intrusions increase the risk for the patient and surgeon. This indication speaks volumes concerning the future medical difficulties a patient may experience. These evidences of body invasion—and the fear that hidden, lingering, destructive alterations need to be considered—haunt prospective surgeons. The accumulated knowledge and skill of the surgeon performing the abdominal repair is crucial. We are becoming more vulnerable with each repeated surgery. The opportunity for securing the best treatment diminishes appreciably the closer we come to being irreparably injured. Minimally invasive procedures that may be available elsewhere ought to be shared with the patient—a standard code of medical ethics should require it.

To the prospective patient I say this: It is so very important to know your surgeon. You must learn about their skill level, which can be ascertained by the number of successful identical surgeries (without complications) they have performed. Earlier I had been critical of the third surgery performance when it became clear that the surgeon himself did not perform the closing procedure. Now you can understand why. That may have diminished my ability to sustain a future attack, or equally important, determined whether I would have had another crisis if the surgeon had performed well. No, just any on-call surgeon or doctor will not do. I'm saying this as a patient with accumulated experience. For a patient, making the assumption that a doctor who is on call has to be good is a terrible mistake. Remember the role concealment plays in the medical profession. It diminishes a patient's ability to establish the quality of the doctor being considered, and the patient cannot make the assumption the hospital has done that.

Given my repeated surgeries, involving in most cases hernia reduction, I was captivated by the success rate of a small hospital outside Toronto, Canada. The distinguishing characteristic was that their surgeons did only hernia surgeries. The normal failure rate, requiring repetitive surgeries, is 10 to 15 percent. This unique hospital's astounding performance was reflected in a failure rate of just 1 percent. The difference here in failure probability is one out of ten versus one out of one hundred. What would you choose for yourself or your family? Dr. Atul Gawande visited the hospital and reported his findings: "I asked Byrnes Shouldice, a son of the founder and a hernia surgeon himself, whether he ever got bored doing hernias all day long. 'No,' he said in a Spock-like voice, 'Perfection is the excitement.'"[30] Variety, embraced by the generalists, may not be the best way to perform many surgeries with perfection. If the incentives reward repetition for failed performance, change will likely come at a snail's pace. Change the incentives and change the performance.

David Goldhill's book, *Catastrophic Care: How American Health Care Killed My Father—and How We Can Fix It,* describes how his eighty-three-year-old father was killed by a sepsis infection he picked up in a hospital while being treated for pneumonia. In an editorial in the *Atlantic*, Mr. Goldhill points out some uncomfortable facts:

> Keeping Dad company in the hospital for five weeks had left me befuddled. How can a facility featuring state-of-the-art diagnostic equipment use less-sophisticated information technology than my local sushi bar? How can the ICU stress the importance of sterility when its trash is picked up once daily, and only after flowing onto the floor of a patient's room? Considering the importance of a patient's frame of mind to recovery, why are the rooms so cheerless and uncomfortable? In whose interest is the bizarre scheduling of hospital shifts, so that a five-week stay brings an endless string of new personnel assigned to a patient's care? Why, in other words, has this technologically advanced hospital missed out on the revolution in quality control and customer service that has swept all other consumer-facing industries in the past two generations?[31]

In the *New York Journal of Books*, reviewer Roberta Winter says:

> Refreshingly, Mr. Goldhill calls for increased transparency in health care services both for pricing and patient safety. Though the Affordable Care Act does mandate more reporting of clinical outcomes, medical supplier pricing, and even insurance company utilization of premium payments, he shows how transparency would impact a health care consumer's decision.

---

[30] Gawande, Complications. p. 39–42.
[31] David Goldhill, "How American Health Care Killed My Father," *Atlantic,* September 2009.

If hospitals were required to post their patient safety scores that alone would help create a level playing field for consumers. Americans currently rely on others to assure their safety, but clearly this method has not proven effective—for us, that is.[32]

I have learned from my own experience that negotiating for medical services is not easy. And finding information about hospital safety is more difficult still. It is helpful to be aware of that.

[32] Roberta E. Winter, "Review of David Goldhill, *Catastrophic Care: How American Health Care Killed My Father—and How We Can Fix It,* (Vintage Press, 2013)," *New York Journal of Books.*

Chapter Thirteen

Surgery Now!

The Clinic scheduled me to meet with their colorectal surgeon on April 12, 2011. Unfortunately, that was a week later than the ticking time bomb of adhesions, hernias, and corresponding blockage would tolerate. I awakened early on the morning of April 5, 2011. The life-threatening symptoms of a blockage were in full custody of my consciousness: severe abdominal pain, vomiting, and chronic hiccups—nothing else mattered. I was forced to enter a local hospital. The diagnosis matched the Clinic's findings, and I was again facing imminent surgery. We called the closest ER and were assured of immediate entry with no delay. Admission was instant, and routine tests performed confirmed the message delivered by the symptoms. Surgery was recommended. I was doubly concerned since I desired the most minimally invasive procedure possible and did not believe I could be assured of that. Because of the urgency I settled for their on-call appointee. The Clinic was consulted and agreed that the risk of transportation and delay was not wise. They knew the level of danger from the CT analysis, which they had completed less than a month earlier.

I felt very fortunate that the gastroenterologist on call was the one we would have selected independently. His reputation for colon care and research was well known to us and the wider medical community.

The investigation indicated a large bowel obstruction from the sigmoid volvulus, all confirming the urgent need for surgery. An attempted colonoscopy to reverse the volvulus was unsuccessful. The risk of perforation, in the judgment of the consulting professionals, necessitated surgery. We consulted with the Clinic, and it was agreed that further delay would be risky.

The official record, dated April 6, 2011, includes these notes in the "Procedure in Detail" section:

> Inspection of the abdomen revealed a colonic volvulus involving the transverse and descending colon. . . . The volvulus occurred around an adhesive band... [adhesions, a gift from repetitive surgeries]. The adhesive band was removed. The volvulus was reduced. . . . Given the clinical situation it was felt the patient was best treated with a temporary colostomy. . . . The patient had multiple defects along the midline from prior surgery. . . . A stoma appliance and sterile dressings were applied. The patient tolerated the procedure well.

Colonic volvulus and ventral hernia reduction were necessary, which in turn left me with a colostomy that prolapsed severely within a few weeks. That complication necessitated an additional surgery.

During my first postoperative meeting with my surgeon, who was exceptionally pleasant and put me at ease, as he inquired, "When are you going to let me put you back together again?" This appeared to be a type of carrot-dangling medical sales pitch. It was coupled with a touch of encouragement for those of us who have suddenly discovered, to our chagrin, we must have our bowel evacuation near the front of our anatomy. It offered a glimmer of hope that I could return to "normal" someday via another surgery, if I survived it and all went as planned. Since my stoma had prolapsed, a serious complication, I had no choice regarding that additional surgery. The rather cavalier comment about putting me back together belied the danger faced in such takedown abdominal surgeries.

These surgeries have not gotten any easier as I continue to rack them up; each requires an eight-inch incision next to the previous scar. The affected tissue multiplies the difficulty level for the surgeon performing the procedure and the risk to the patient. Each one prolongs the time required for recovery. I delayed the next surgery to enable me to gain at least ten pounds, keenly aware of surgery's toll on my recovery and the risk to my life. The fifth surgery, described below, involved "unconventional" intestinal maneuvering to reconnect (takedown) and restore "normal" bowel functions. I chose the surgeon who performed the emergency surgery in April of 2011 because of his direct knowledge of my condition and the excellent relationship we had developed. We were also eager to have the same gastroenterologist for the reasons listed above. We delayed the procedure a couple of weeks so he would be available to perform the colonoscopy required prior to surgery. (He is also my current choice for follow-up care now that I have recovered from the surgeries. He has been very helpful in offering guidance for monitoring my bowel functions.)

My medical record from September 22, 2011, states:

Procedure in Detail. The abdominal cavity was entered without difficulty. . . . Extensive adhesiolyosis [severing of adhesive bands, again] was undertaken. The stoma was located in the left upper quadrant. This was dissected free from the surrounding structures. The colon was divided at the level of the peritoneum [the membrane that lines the wall of the abdominal cavity] with the contour stapler. . . . It was slightly dilated. . . . The small bowel was freed from ligament of Treitz [a band of muscle from the junction of the duodenum jejunum to the left crus of the diaphragm, a suspensory ligament] . . . with extensive adhesiolyosis. . . . Due to the patient's known volvulus it was decided to perform a cecopexy [which anchors the cecum to the abdominal wall]. . . . The patient tolerated the procedure well.

I had accepted an on-call (rotating) surgeon in this blocked-bowel emergency. The credential of comfort he had was an internship at the avant-garde medical institution (the previously discussed renowned Clinic). I had scheduled my follow-up there based on their CT scan, which had correctly indicated a blockage was imminent. It is often difficult to enlist quality surgeons to treat a compromised surgical patient, for the reasons I have already shared. However, in this case, the surgeon who performed this latest procedure turned out to be just what I needed. He was always available, and generous with his time and expertise, when we felt a need to consult.

Opinion of an Experienced Patient

I have an observation regarding the assertion that abdominal surgery should be performed by general surgeons. The complexity of the abdominal area and the risks of complications from infection and latent adhesion formation with invasive procedures should merit the expertise of highly specialized and gifted surgeons whose skill is derived in part from numerous repetitions. I make no attempt here to detract from the skill of the generalist, but repetition improves performance. Recall the excellent record of the hospital that performed only hernia surgeries?[33]

Some progressive clinics have begun to label procedures such as colorectal surgery, which is highly specific and, if possible, minimally invasive, as standard practice, but for many reasons it is not. I now

---

[33]   Gawande, Complications p. 39–42.

suffer from several eight-inch abdominal scars and lumpy hernia protrusions that may not continue functioning without additional attention. Patients deserve the best possible results, but the incentives for providing this seem to be missing. The general surgeon, on average, may be less skillful in producing the stellar results, since precise repetition appears to significantly enhance performance, even given the general surgeon's overall talent. So when it comes time to choose a surgeon to perform your operation, make sure you choose someone who has significant *proven* skills. It is your life—don't ever forget it. Remember, too, that this is a nonprofessional's point of view.

Abdominal Overview from an Experienced Surgeon

The abdominal area seems especially challenging, according to Dr. Paul Ruggieri, chief of the department of surgery at a large, Eastern community hospital. He states matter-of-factly:

> I often cringe when I find a long abdominal scar on a patient I need to operate on. Previous surgery creates scar tissue, which in turn makes my job inside and outside the operating room more difficult. In addition to increasing the risk of 'collateral' damage inside the operating room, previous surgery can lead to prolonged recovery time in the hospital. What are Mr. Andrews' chances of surviving if the operation does not go perfectly?[34]

You will become better acquainted with Dr. Ruggieri later in the book (Chapter Eighteen, Applied Medical Mythology) as he relates an actual abdominal surgery he performed on a patient as an on-call general surgeon. I can say at this point it may give one pause

---

[34] Paul A. Ruggieri, *Confessions of a Surgeon* (New York: Berkley Publishing Group, 2012). p. 57.

regarding what lurks below those abdominal scars—he is certainly in a position to know.

I write this beyond the one-year anniversary of my fifth surgery. It was more than a year ago and seems, via the passage of time, even more distant. But this incision, inflicted upon previous incisions—upon incisions upon incisions upon incisions—has still not fully healed. While I was recuperating, there were many problems that could have created more difficulties.

I have been under the supervision of a wound-care center affiliated with the hospital where I received the most recent surgery. Some who examined me at times touched the wound area without gloves; the waiting facilities were at times unhygienic in appearance, and the wait durations were sometimes up to an hour. When I expressed my own frustration with the very tender skin around the surgical area, one medical clinician helped educate me: "Mr. Huber, at the very best your skin can only return to 80 percent of its original strength." That was the first time I recall hearing that. The doctor, nurses, and receptionists were always very kind and helpful with any problem I brought to their attention. I have the utmost gratitude for their dedication in this demanding and vital service.

As I write, I am still battling a healing difficulty complicated by the MRSA infection I contracted during my second surgery (the one meant to undo damage inflicted from complications via the original robotic procedure). You're never free of MRSA. My terribly disfigured abdominal profile is now distended due to multiple hernias. I am now past the second month's regimen of antibiotics (doxycycline hyclate) as well as daily dressing changes performed with assistance from my dedicated wife. It is difficult to wear any abdominal support or fasten my seatbelt because the tender and still-fragile skin cannot sustain the compression without further damage.

As I keep reminding my readers (it's no small matter), I have borne the total cost of this grueling medical marathon, which began in November 2007. A systemic change is a must, and some very highly credentialed representatives of this distinguished profession, as quoted in this treatise, are coming forward and openly sharing their concerns and recommendations. Many of these directives are listed here for you.

My own small voice is being added to balance the feedback with the patient's account; medical professionals are supported with the confirming voices of their patients.

I returned to the Clinic in February 2013 for an evaluation of my present status and to keep my list of contacts current in case I had another emergency. The colorectal surgeon I had been referred to in April 2011 has retired. After a careful examination he referred me to other specialists who would follow up on my case should I encounter difficulties in the future. Below I share a portion of my medical record, written by an abdominal surgeon in residence there. His assessment of my condition, dated February 4, 2013, is as follows:

He has healed skin on his abdominal wall but basically has skin on bowel, the consequence of healing by granulation. . . . He has approximate 8 cm. defect at costal margin and a 15 cm musculofascial effect at his umbilicus. . . . I could not get his thin skin on his upper abdomen to stretch to the midline. On attempted Valsalva, he cannot lift the shoulders off the table and does not medialize his rectus muscles with a forced Valsalva [a procedure performed by attempting to forcibly exhale while keeping the mouth and nose closed].

Assessment/Plan

The surgeon in residence continued:

Mr Huber should avoid any elective operation. The fact that his skin has healed on his abdominal wall is excellent for him. . . . I do not recommend any hernia surgery because tissue coverage will be an issue as he has immobile rectus muscles and some lateral incisions, which would preclude rectus muscle mobilization and very poor skin.

In our extended conversation with the reputable surgeon, he volunteered an opinion I deem rare in the medical profession. He stated that I should not permit any of those responsible for my abdominal condition to perform any further surgeries on me—one surgeon's opinion in retrospect. An earlier report cited a pelvic-floor dysfunction. Floors and doors that are out of sync create problems for the patient, making it difficult to produce normal bowel movements. It was determined that my rectal signaling process was opposite what it should be. The force applied in attempting a bowel movement created the reverse physiological response, precluding the desired action.

This reminds me of a poem I saw on a trinket in a shopping mall. "Doors marked pull reduce the speed of those who push before they read." Not something you want pasted on your bathroom mirror—but whatever works.

New Certification Rules

A recent *Wall Street Journal* article by journalist Laura Landro discussed controversial new certification requirements being mandated for doctors in order for them to stay current with rapidly changing medical advances.[35] As Landro explains:

> Doctors were once board-certified for life, but in the 1970s some boards began to issue time-limited certificates. Dr. Baron says physicians certified by his board before 1990 will remain certified for life but will be reported as "not meeting requirements" if they don't participate in maintenance activities.

The need to qualify a doctor or surgeon is becoming understood by the medical community, and they are organizing to improve doctors' performance. In addition, they're working to make that information available to patients who are justifiably wary of the attitude that just any doctor will do. As we have stated repeatedly, the medical profession's standard is to overstate the abilities of their professionals to the degree that the members themselves adopt that persona and as a result may become threats to patients. Imagine certifying a professional for life. *What were they thinking?*

As Landro explains in her article:

> Studies show clinical skills deteriorate over time and doctor's overconfidence can lead to diagnostic errors. A 2006 review in the Journal of the American Medical Association found that doctors aren't very good at evaluating their own skills. University of Michigan professor R. Van Harrison, an author of the study, says maintenance of certification "is part of a larger evolution of the health-care system." He says big hospital systems are helping doctors meet certification requirements as part of larger quality-improvement programs.

---

[35]   Laura Landro, "How Qualified Is Your Doctor? Doctors Face New Requirements to Keep Up-to-Date to Stay Certified," *Wall Street Journal*, January 20, 2014.

Insert yourself into my picture. Scan through five surgeries in as many years. Now contemplate what is fair and just in the distribution of accountability. Your conclusion may be similar to that of many critical professionals now speaking out. Many are convinced only transparency can bring us to the reckoning table.

THE HUBER FAMILY

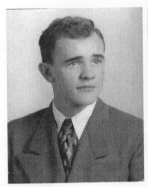 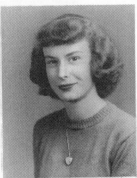

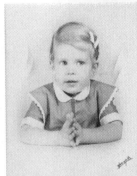 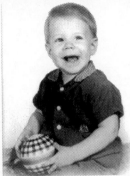 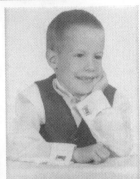

George Huber, Ella Mae Huber, children: Rebecca
Huber, Brent Huber, and Bart Huber

It is reminiscent of sitting for a family photo. The kids and adults become equally impatient needing to appear to be something we'll never achieve. The ever present intuition and consciousness is within before we can even comprehend it. We have a galactocentric future, the telescope's gift, not an ordinary past-dominated vision via the rearview mirror. Especially with the heavens attractions, coming now to Earth's tiny theatre, there is the subtle awareness that we are looking deeply into revealed stellar history of space and time. Before memory's echo of the experience falls silent, the landscape, our little piece of terra firma, has changed dramatically. Toddlers, who could not sit still, have made their mark, and the adults, the only authority, by nature have vanished from the scene. The future's important discoveries will provide clues to questions we do not yet know how to ask, and will prelude innovations no one could ever predict or imagine.

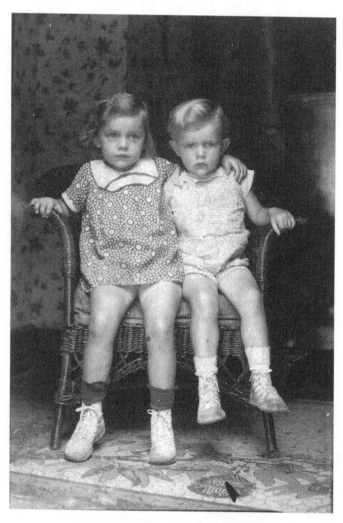

KID SISTER AND BROTHER

Kid sister and brother, Honey and Buddy (monikers we still use), busily helping each other grow up. We were younger by a couple of decades compared to our older three sisters and two brothers. That separation, nearly generational, made Honey and me very close.

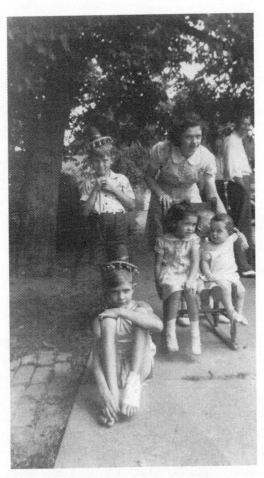

BICYCLE ENCOUNTER

My thirty-pound bicycle defied a 3000 pound auto. A rear wheel of the car came to rest atop my little foot. We had an excellent surgical outcome, but were still removing pieces of gravel three to six months hence. Some members of our delightful family are present, my sister Agnes Huber Ellis and three daughters, Janice, Jean, and Judy, along with a neighborhood friend.

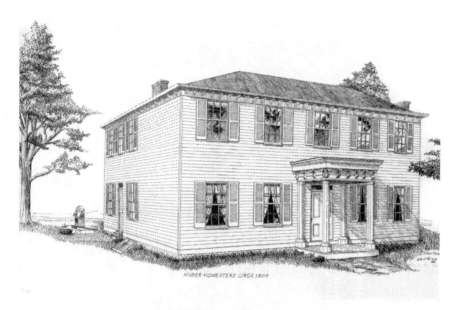

HUBER HOMESTEAD CIRCA 1900

HUBER HOMESTEAD

The Huber Homestead was impressive and located well beyond the angry river's reach. This large, elegant structure was built by our ancestors prior to the Civil War and remained in the family until it became party to an estate sale in the late 1960s. It was enjoyably spacious. This graceful, nine-room edifice would have been the envy of most modern structures in the area. It had an incredible customized organ, designed especially for that house and the spirit and temperament of our heirs, and entertained several generations. This image was drawn from memory by the artistically talented great-great-great-grandson, William Rorick. Judging from my memory, having visited on numerous occasions as a child, he has given the family an incredibly accurate resemblance. We are indebted to Mr. Rorick for each of the artistic reproductions depicted here. I am deeply indebted to the inspiration of my late sister, Della Huber Rorick, the artist's mother, for the pithy historical information in this narrative, and inspiring and encouraging the artistic memory of our numerous generations.

AN IMMIGRANT'S CONTRIBUTION

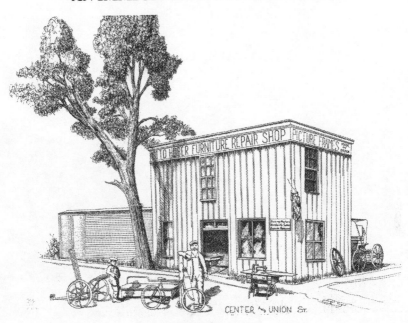

OTTO HUBER

Otto Huber, whose rustic business shop, as represented here, was a resident in the family home in the early 1900s. This is a vivid example of the spirit of thrift and creativity brought to our shores by those we learned to first tolerate, then accept, and finally respect for their valued contributions. They were quite good at seeing a need, providing a service, and earning their place here. William Rorick, artist.

RAMPAGING RIVER

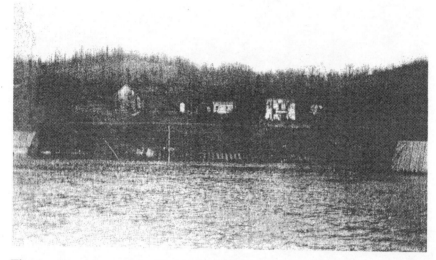

The two-story house in which I was born and reared is depicted with just the slightest apex of the roof visible, as though gasping for air, just above the water, taken during the epic 1937 flood. Many dwellings did not survive it, as you see on the next page.

RIVER FOLKS—ALWAYS BEGIN AGAIN

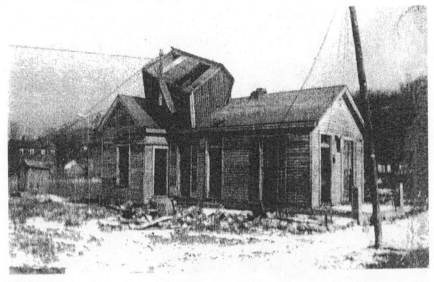

Being a child of the Ohio River Valley, I am not in the least surprised by the poetic mythology that anthropomorphizes a river's influence and at times gives meaning to the domination it has over our lives. Some intrusions have been so catastrophic as to be life altering. I request your indulgence here as I have included a few dramatic images that were life changing for me and my family as I was growing up, and for many others as well. River people will easily understand that proximity and elevation are calculated risks on the river—and there are staggering consequences.

FIRST FERRY

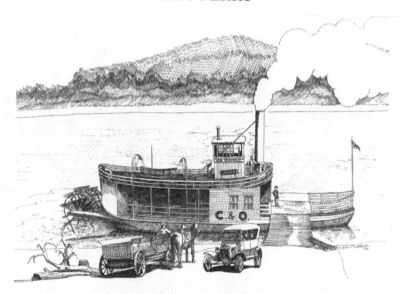

NEW RICHMOND FERRY 1912

FERRY

Every river needs a ferry, and New Richmond's very earliest is shown here. It was used primarily for passengers and light cargo and was vital for social connections to our neighboring sister state of Kentucky. William Rorick, artist.

OPERA HOUSE 1874-1957

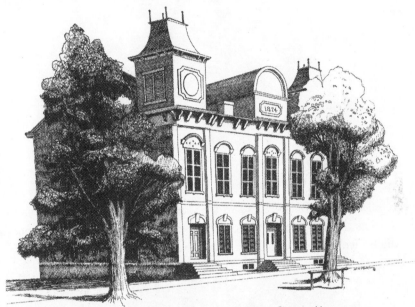

OHIO TOWNSHIP HALL — OPERA HOUSE ~
POST OFFICE, NEW RICHMOND, O. 1874~1957

On the literary scene, a touch of elegance, the community's delightful
opera house has been represented for us. This legendary, classical facility,
a perfect venue reminiscent of dances, fairs, plays, and modest oratorios,
an historical tribute to our small community. William Rorick, artist.

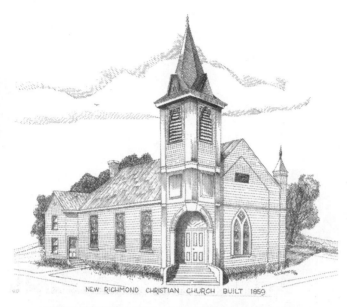

NEW RICHMOND CHRISTIAN CHURCH

The church was built in 1859 and we worshiped there as children. It has been artistically rendered here as well by William Rorick. That is the church in which I was ordained into the ministry as depicted below.

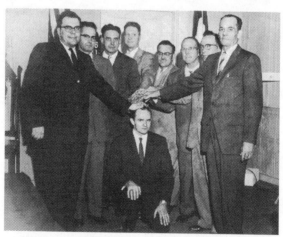

ORDINATION

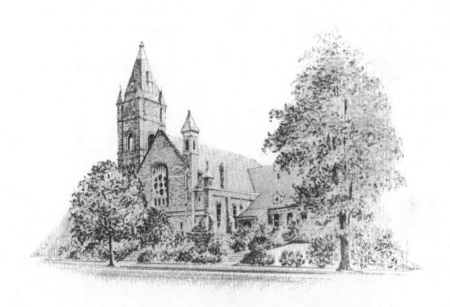

CINCINNATI CHRISTIAN UNIVERSITY

SEMINARY CHAPEL

The seminary chapel where I had the honor of participating and worshiping during the years I studied there in the 1950s.

IN MEMORY OF MY MENTORS

Any achievements I have experienced I must share with the creators of inspiration and counsel from which I have benefited immensely. My strength in educational pursuits came from two vital encounters with the most talented men I have ever met. Good fortune smiled on me early in having these two remarkably gifted and generous mentors during my early educational, religious and social endeavors in academic communities.

MENTOR NUMBER ONE

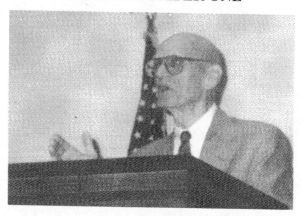

Dr. Lewis Foster

Dr. Lewis Foster (BD, Yale Divinity School; STM, Harvard Divinity School; PhD in history and philosophy of religion, Harvard School of Arts and Sciences) was a professor and mentor whose instruction I treasure. I was privileged to enroll in his classes while pursuing my ThB, and thereafter I frequently sought his counsel in founding a campus student ministry for members of our denomination as they pursued their studies at Miami University of Ohio.

MENTOR NUBMER TWO

DR. ROY WARD

Dr. Roy Ward, Bachelor of Sacred Theology (STB) and Doctor of Theology (ThD 1967) from Harvard University. He became Professor of Comparative Religion and later Associate Provost at Miami University, Oxford, Ohio. His career began in 1964. Dr. Ward, upon hearing of our student religious foundation there, contacted me, and asked if he could join us in this endeavor. He and I worked together on this important program until I left to continue my studies at the University of Florida.

MIAMI UNIVERSITY SEQUICENTENNIAL CHAPEL

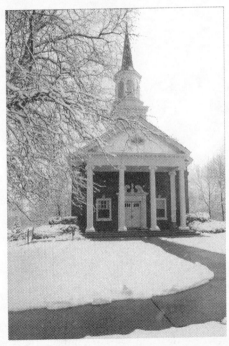

The beautiful Sesquicentennial Chapel on the campus of Miami University in Oxford, Ohio, where I had the pleasure of officiating marriage rites for several student couples. It represented for them the beginning of a shared life. Now their education really began in earnest.

ECHOES OF TENNIS PAST

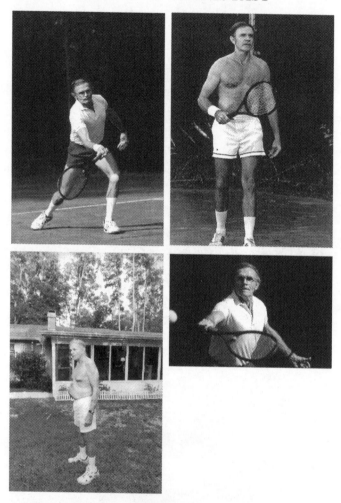

TENNIS PHOTOS (George Huber)

My tennis photos are contrasted with that of the medically induced distended abdomen. "Before and After" are consequences of surgical complications that went terribly wrong. I was a fitness enthusiast; I enjoyed intense physical activity and relished good health. My discipline was no match for error-prone medicals. I was destined for a life-altering trauma; the unexpected and dramatic diminution of life as I had come to know it. That surgery ended my cherished tennis pursuit, my hobby of choice. I am still struggling with the abdominal dilation after five such surgeries, performed as they were, thus producing this obvious outcome. This is by no means a call for sympathy, but an admonitory alert.

Chapter Fourteen

Enter Transparency

You can observe a lot by just watching.

—Yogi Berra

The medical system has been engaged in a longstanding and negative pattern of concealing complications—failed surgeries—repeatedly denying responsibility for injuring, maiming, and yes, even killing patients. To solve the problem of these hidden issues, a powerful antidote has been summoned: transparency. If this were a novel, our two principal characters would be transparency and accountability. You will find them inserting themselves at every hint of injustice or unfairness; their roles are played conjointly.

Those following financial and political corruption will know that a similar remedy has been prescribed for those institutions too. As we have seen, these traditional systems are reacting as expected—with a protective fervor. Concealment represents a systemic effort to maintain stability with the existing structure; and it regards change as alien. Openness on the other hand contributes to their enhancement in an evolving science by sharing the evaluative process with a larger community and inviting new ideas. The protective fear is that openness and disclosure will cause incalculable harm. Medicine as a life science is energized by the light of openness; better ideas eagerly await an invitation to serve. Secrecy is stifling and antithetical to the goals of a progressive system. This evaluative dimension of transparency is new to medicine and will need to make peace with personal privacy and the generational conflicts.

The positive side is also consistent with our democratic principles. The more people know, the more they support fairness, justice, and equality and the more insistent they are that their institutions live up to their stated commitments and be held accountable. Most of us believe that, when we confront injustice and unfairness, silence akin to that maintained by the medical community crosses the line of fairness and the patient suffers. Transparency is an incentive for our leaders to administer our institutions with integrity and be rewarded for their service. Keep in mind medical institutions are political too.

The old-school political truism asserting that what you say is more important than what you do will join the mound of discarded sophistry. Transparency has become one of the more highly successful strategies as we formulate the goals and monitor the performance of our fundamental institutions. Listen carefully, and you will hear it paired with accountability; they progress in tandem.

Chapter Fifteen

Primordial Origins of Dysfunctional Systems

Horns, Halos, and Happenstance

Measuring the functionality of a system requires assessing overall performance and projecting future outcomes. Since we have alleged ethical compromises and failures, with resulting life and death consequences, cultural value vetting emerges. Fundamentally we will start at the most elementary level: Is it good or bad?

Good versus evil, as a values metric may not be as helpful as traditionally presumed. It triggers collective memory in a polarizing way. Given the vast symbolic stigma and the subsequent bias attached, little objective social merit is derived from it. Ignorance is seldom explicitly factored in but plays a heretofore unrecognized role in this design. Awareness of the time factor in cultural evolution is crucial. The earth used to be flat, and we behaved differently. What was regarded as righteous indignation (good) by our ancestor's assessment during the Middle Ages is considered horribly barbaric today. Attempts to parse inhumanity as applicable across cultures in current societies demonstrate the incongruence of historic barbarism forwarded and activated in modern societies. The current adoption of ancient aggression via raw power is a violation of modern international standards. Conquests undertaken according to those obsolete standards, regardless of numerous historic examples, are primitive to us and are now regarded as criminal. Appealing to ancestral or ancient precedents, sacred or secular, carries less influence in the world court of global judgment. We are making progress, slowly.

We are all members of communities organized by systems on which we depend. The world, the USA, the states and municipalities in which we live, our neighborhoods, the organizations for which we work, our families and others are contributing components. Authentic systemic approaches, where governing systems prevail, such as nationalism, democracy, socialism, secularism, communism, feudalism, and tribalism, are operating amid varied mixtures—hybrids of these structures. Intolerance, tolerance, and acceptance are on a recognizable continuum. Inclusion and acceptance of communities, welcoming differences from cultures, languages, and heritages, thereby facilitating boundary integration and dissolving hostility, are worthy but difficult goals not yet universally recognized. This much we should agree on: societies and systems based on lies are destined to fail, regardless of the stature of the fabricators.

Our systems control us, and religious institutions in a democracy must navigate a fine line to prevent the entanglement of church and state. Wisdom is vindicated as the unspeakable treachery and manipulative abuses, past and present, unfold repeatedly under religious intolerance and inquisitions. A personal incident is relevant here: My wife and I were watching a bit of filler TV on one occasion a few years ago. The famed film *The Godfather*, still quite popular, was being shown. I watched for less than a half hour and said, "Honey, there is just too much violence for me—sorry." I went to the study and resumed my reading. At the time, I was reviewing *A History of Christianity* by Kenneth Scott Latourette, Sterling professor of Missions and Oriental history, and fellow of Berkeley College at

Yale University.[36] I just so happened to be in a section covering the religious wars. The chapter was entitled "Repudiation and Revival, A.D. 1750—A.D. 1815." It recounted Voltaire and Hume, among others, and depicted the endless violence for heretical cleansing during that period. In less than an hour, I rejoined my wife with the comment, "There is less violence in what you are watching than in what I am reading!"

In our democratic society I believe we are most fortunate that religion is not authorized to rule.

Humankind's sectarian history is rife with systems provoking incidents in which killing thy neighbor is advocated as the solution to resolve conflicts, when authoritarian edicts, both religious and secular, are imposed and collide with cultural differences that lack resolution. These incidents aggravate exponentially the conflicts they purport to resolve. The garment of basic civility is rent asunder, and the demon latent in political systems erupts and wreaks havoc through both religious and secular manipulation, to influence and to win allegiance and loyalty for its myriad causes. In the pursuit of power, there is seldom a balanced, democratic blend. However, authoritarian regimes may find even that totally incompatible.

When religion is summoned as sovereign, a preferred paradigm of endorsed succession for the anointed adherents is invoked.

An unbroken string connecting past to present is a stratagem employed frequently by religious authorities, to legitimize a government's pursuits, with the idea that they have an implicit right to prevail in controversies by imposing power while subverting reasoned discourse. Revered leaders, often professing thousands of

---

[36]   Kenneth Scott Latourette, A History of Christianity, New York, Harper Brothers, 1953. p. 1001-1059

years of continuous endorsement, are depicted as chosen heirs with a divine right certified and validated on the basis of their appeal to ancient sacred texts. Myths abound, but there are rules, even here, that must be observed for the system to function.

Anything written is representational; therefore, it must be interpreted. By the very nature of symbolic communication, nothing can be taken literally. Contextual assessment and consistency are essential. Julius Caesar should not be depicted motoring about the streets of Rome in a jeep. There is room here for the science of linguistics, where it is tolerated.

Assignment of authority to a prescribed tradition or deity on that premise seems very fragile if reason is to prevail. Further imposing a given interpretation on others to justify and enforce power will result in an endless struggle for dominance. One not initiated in these traditions is likely to be puzzled and perplexed by the ascendance of such presumed authorities on that foundation. In controversies, their subjective premise is authenticated—usually derived from cherry-picked quotations of a text echoing from the distant past, the older the better, as chronological distance complicates precise analysis. In a quest for truth, remoteness is inversely proportional to confidence in the applicability of analysis.

It is naïve at best to anticipate civil outcomes by invoking such traditions and imposing behavioral certainties. Rivers of blood have been spilled over these pretexts, interpretations, and dogmas. How many angels can dance on the head of a pin? What sacred real estate or geographical boundary can be determined to have been forever deified in that isolated and distant past? Who are the current legitimate heirs? When we describe this procedure without attributing specific identifying labels, it is clearly and unspeakably irrational. The consequences can be catastrophic. How could we expect otherwise? Men, women, and children are slaughtered. Millions are displaced, as they flee for their lives fearing imminent genocide for alleged lack of racial or ethnic purity or for having trespassed some obscure but strictly imposed fanatical edict. Killing others in the name of some procrustean tradition, shrouded in antiquity, makes no sense unless rituals have become realities by continuous repetition, not by reason. These actions suppress, uproot, and replace rational thought, and incite and justify inhumane treatment in a nonnegotiable intolerance.

Our fragile world cannot continue perpetrating such hoaxes in the name of voracious and vengeful deities. Heirs, claiming legitimacy from endorsement by the lawmaker of the universe, are difficult or impossible to confirm. Select groups divine and extrapolate rules regarding the minutest functions of daily life, exacting vengeance on those who misunderstand, or dare doubt or disagree. Most such rituals and regulations hearken back to a time when the earth was flat, and man the center of the universe.

Having moved through the anthropocentric, geocentric, heliocentric, and galactocentric replicas, we now have lots to contemplate. Such systems are strained to say the least, and in order for tyrants to prevail, they must become enforcers. Having graduated from stones, spears, bows, and arrows to nuclear potential, conscious deliberation has become a must.

We, as members of the human race, with pockets of primitive principles and high-tech destructive power, may not survive with so little time to grow up. The future languishes while so many are mired in that phantom of certainties heralding from the distant past. It is always remote enough that certifiable evidence cannot be presented and a fanatical certainty is urged and embraced to snuff out any conceivable qualms regarding cherished dogmas. If our quest is truth, this contradictory maze of confusion cannot all be true.

It Is the System We Challenge

In this manuscript, I have deliberately chosen not to identify a single group or geographical boundary. That would preclude our thinking about the ramifications of such systems. It is the system we challenge. Simply believing in something, wanting it to be true, or fantasizing that it is true will not make it so. Only firm evidence in support of facts leads to truth—from astrology to astronomy, alchemy to chemistry, enchanted potions to modern medicine, magic to science. The culprit, the inhuman social plague, is the mass of calcified rituals morphed into reality by endless reiteration, beyond any semblance of reason. I repeat, I am not targeting or referring to any specific persons, groups, or places. This is a description of systems. If no such entities described here exist on our planet, ignore this as a frivolous fiction. If they do, we do know they have no place in a functioning, civilized society and will wreak devastation in any attempted social order. Perpetual chaos will ensue; that is their destiny.

This is such a deadly social virus that, were I physically present under its wake, any hint of a challenge would be regarded as a potentially fatal infection; such a threat would be destroyed, lest it spread. Any intruder's life would be in danger under the charges of treason, heresy, or sacrilege. Thoughts alone in such systems would be enough to elicit condemnation. One would have rudely trespassed and exposed the favorite tools of abusive, corruptive power and authority while in fervent denial of doing so. In order for this dynamic to work effectively, it should be employed surreptitiously and deceptively as modernity approaches.

The denial is cemented in the repudiation that the conveyance of one's position has been derived symbolically through interpretation, which is in fact an evaluative conclusion. It is a symbolic conveyance riding on the wheels of interpretation.

I recall once seeing a cartoon (whose source I have been unsuccessful in obtaining) that depicted a person seated before a desk during a job interview. The interviewer comments, "I notice here that you have stated your long-term goal is world conquest." Flash back a few millennia and that might have been a quite laudable declaration. In fact it was the quintessence of Alexander the Great's every activity. Timing has much to do with systemic reality. The problem with literalists is that antiquated cultural norms get intertwined with sacred texts and obfuscate the spiritual message that is in fact timeless.

The messenger here, in a crude way, has become a systemic whistleblower in the challenge. That is hardly a comfortable role to play given the nature of these systems.

Failed systems need to be examined and evaluated. Peter Ludlow recently laid out criteria for our consideration. The title of his article is piercing and direct, "The Banality of Systemic Evil." Systems can and do go bad for some of the reasons stated above. When they do, we have to make significant corrections. That requires assistance from within and without; only then can we trust our systems to provide the anticipated service in the most comprehensive and effective way. He writes:

Here is a moral principle at work in the actions of the leakers, whistle-blowers and hacktivists and those who support them. I would also argue that that moral principle has been clearly articulated, and it may just save us from a dystopian future. . . . Similarly it is possible that the system itself is sick, even though the actors within the organization are behaving in accord with organizational protocol and respecting the internal bonds of trust.

For the leaker and whistleblower . . . there can be no expectation that the system will act morally of its own accord. Systems are optimized for their own survival and preventing the system from doing evil may well require breaking with organizational niceties, protocols or laws. It requires stepping outside of one's assigned organizational role. The chief executive is not in a better position to recognize systemic evil than is a middle level manager or, for that matter, an IT contractor. Recognizing systemic evil does not require rank or intelligence, just honesty of vision.[37]

The art of progress is to preserve order amid change, and to preserve change amid order.

—Alfred North Whitehead,

mathematician and philosopher (1861–1947)

Carl Sagan, the scientist who needs little introduction, gave a graphic description of the failure of such systems to advance us to a level of mutual acceptance and compassion for our fellow humans:[38]

The Earth is a very small stage in a vast cosmic arena. Think of the rivers of blood spilled by all those generals and emperors so that, in glory and triumph, they could become the momentary masters of a fraction of a dot. Think of the endless cruelties visited by the inhabitants of one corner of this pixel on the scarcely distinguishable inhabitants of some other corner, how frequent their misunderstandings, how eager they are to kill one another, how fervent their hatreds.

---

[37] Peter Ludlow, "The Banality of Systemic Evil," Opinionator. *New York Times*, September 15, 2013.

[38] Carl Sagan, (1997) Pale Blue Dot: A Vision of the Human Future in Space, retrieved from:
http://www.goodreads.com/work/quotes/1816628-pale-blue-dot-a-vision-of-the-human-future-in-space

Chapter Sixteen

Trusting Citizens

What, when, where, by whom, for what purpose, and under what circumstances shall information under the auspices of our institutions be disclosed or withheld from citizens? National attention was captivated with the alleged security breaches surrounding the recent whistleblower scandals such as that involving former NSA employee Edward Snowden and others. They focused passionate debate on the role of government in rationing information-sharing while privatizing our nation's security structure—a transparency-versus-opacity issue that is of great concern. The results will require prolonged moral, ethical, political, and legal battles before the dust settles, even temporarily. We should not permit that to obfuscate the role transparency will play increasingly in the strength and vigor of our social, financial, medical, educational, and governmental institutions. While their influence may be overrated at times, that influence has been summoned for assistance in battling corruption on multiple fronts. We are learning from our mistakes, and secrecy may not always protect a wholesome endeavor.

The charge that revealing such histories violates security should be vetted, verified, and validated by designated bipartisan and objective representatives rather than left to the designs of a prejudicial, political, and overly protective partisan bias. On issues where citizens have been consistently misled or misinformed this demonstrates our democracy's need for accurate and timely information to guarantee quality decisions assured by transparency and accountability. That is the road to a more mature and responsible citizenry and more effective institutions and government. The challenge to such disclosures have often been security based and labeled excessively as unpatriotic—even criminal. Hyping dangers to our national unity has been shown, not infrequently, to be a cover for political incompetence and a maneuver to avoid embarrassment.

No Harm Street, Wall Street, and Main Street comprise the important pillars of our society. They have all been impacted negatively by this tendency to overstress the need for secrecy under the guise of essential institutional protection. What citizens need assurance of is that the quest for nondisclosure is legitimate and doesn't represent a shield from embarrassing failed policies and practices to help institutions avoid accountability. A standing bipartisan council should oversee this process and prevent nonessential restrictions. The people need to know, and good government—an orchestra of systems—will become even better government with that incentive, the awareness that the people will know. On No Harm Street, concealment has been systemic, and has also undermined patient fairness, and denied and deflected judgment to prevent accountability. Democratic precautions must have our people as fully informed as possible on all three streets.

Our Government Consists of People Too

The greater the gap between the middle and lower classes from the elite financial echelon, who influence governance, the further removed they are from honest disclosure and interaction, the more dysfunctional they become. The drastic rise over the past few decades in extreme wealth disparity creates an insidious shield by isolating those at the top from day-to-day transparency essential for cultivating empathy. It creates gross inequality, and the effect is a polarizing of the institutions in our society, which results in their withdrawal to areas that they control and that are separate from their life experiences. The governors should know the life of the governed and feel genuine compassion for them. Whether this is intended or not (i.e., due to willful isolation or just insensitivity from lack of exposure), they seem out of touch with the multitudes whose lives are impacted by lobbied decisions that exclude them. We seem to have forgotten that our government is people too.

Steven Greenhouse, who reports on labor issues for the New York Times and is author of *The Big Squeeze: Tough Times for the American Worker*, reported in the *Times*:

> "We went almost a century where the labor share was pretty stable and we shared prosperity," says Lawrence Katz, a labor economist at Harvard. "What we're seeing now is very disquieting." For the great bulk of workers, labor's shrinking share is even worse than the statistics show, when one considers that a sizable—and growing— chunk of overall wages goes to the top 1 percent: senior corporate executives, Wall Street professionals, Hollywood stars, pop singers and professional athletes. The share of wages going to the top 1 percent climbed to 12.9 percent in 2010, from 7.3 percent in 1979.[39]

Born on Third Base—Heritable Celebrities

An "unearned triple," or an educational elitism dubbed a "legacy," which I prefer, has become another institutionalized mechanism of note, as it dramatically favors wealthy contributors to select Ivy League universities as the price for assuring their heirs

---

[39] Steven Greenhouse, "Our Economic Pickle," *New York Times*, January 13, 2013.

entry into those hallowed halls under a tailored academic standard, purchased by the influence of inherited wealth. Buying access to many institutions has become too customary to avoid hurting our democracy and consequently our nation. Our country bears the scars of leaders selected based on heredity over competence. Consequently, colleges are becoming a fixed class system disingenuously marketed. They are unavailable to most applicants, accessible instead only to the insiders. In the medical world, there is favoritism in health services at an elevated level also reserved for the elite. Legacy has engendered a humorous ruse: Individuals "born on third base,"—and for the more obtuse benefactors, "Yes, and they thought they just hit a triple!" They show up as a subject without a predicate. Therein lies a danger—self-deception, compounded by such imperceptive incompetence and inadequate performance. They are unprepared to pass through opportunities' gates, but they can and do, and then inflict lasting harm before multiple tragic outcomes turn them away. Or, as we have heard more than a few times, especially in politics they believe, "It's my turn!" Talent must be the dominating factor, yes, and even then, there is a lot of luck needed to boot.

Such an academic rite of passage as a gatekeeper to power reeks of signature elitism, regardless of universities' contention that they could not maintain their plush endowments without it. Better forfeit them when such endowments influence both the welfare of our country and the world. Honor and power bestowed, yet unearned, bring with them a host of negative consequences.

That open door for those of inherited wealth is obviously closed to some more talented and deserving by that very fact. This is just another means for advantageous treatment that widens the gap between the haves and have-nots, or between insiders and outsiders, which as we have seen has serious social, financial, medical, and cultural implications. I could catalog examples endlessly to substantiate our abandonment of a real semblance of equality. We don't all play by the same rules. We don't all share equal opportunities. The rules are written with well-lobbied intentions; favoritism is signed, sealed, and delivered, yet we recoil at more penetrating designations such as "legalized bribery." Instead of a royal family we have a score of "royal" inherited legacies "crowned" by excess wealth, taking when they should be giving, awarded in the absence of merit, diluting excellence, and destined to fall to their level of incompetence, dispensing disaster in their wake. This is relevant, as we shall see, on all fronts and especially as we envision a medical democracy. We can't apply enough whitewash to euphemize our way out of this.

Lessons from the Sixties

A leading social and political critic, Allan Bloom, in his epic book *The Closing of the American Mind*, challenges us in ways that few teachers have. His knowledge of history and philosophy are unsurpassed by estimation of the leading critics of his day. Given the esoteric caliber of his subject, it is amazing that it remained a best-seller for the latter part of the 1980s. Dealing extensively with the universities of the sixties, the book captured my interest and admiration. No subject was off limits. I wish to call your attention to his assessment of the university and its values vacuum. I remember the sixties well from my own experience on the university campus. For those wondering what in the world this has to do with medicine, you only need ask where we get our doctors, nurses, and pharmacists? Bloom feared for the survival of those institutions dependent on a disintegrating educational system. We're back to systems again.

Bloom was keenly aware of our tendency to have a very short attention span and interest index even for very important issues. He knew how easily our society could be riveted on a problem, be it natural disaster; a gun rampage by a deranged, mentally ill misfit; abuse of minorities; or controversy surrounding public education. He offered this delicate little jewel as a reminder: "Forgetting, in a variety of subtle forms, is one of our primary modes of problem-solving."

Comparing American and German universities, he warns:

> The university had abandoned all claim to study or inform about value—undermining the sense of the value of what it taught, while turning over the decision about values to the folk, the Zeitgeist, the relevant. . . . As Hegel was said to have died in Germany in 1933, Enlightenment in America came close to breathing its last during the sixties.[40]

That was the period in which social upheaval spread to the university campus. The rebellion in response to the Vietnam War challenged all our institutions. Bloom's loathing of mobs taking the university hostage stemmed from his recognition that it was antithetical to the purpose of the university. Community interaction for conflict resolution was an important role of the university. Deliberative intellectual engagement was a means of achieving civility and harmony—the end of barbarism.

I have chosen Bloom's treatises from that era to demonstrate the necessity for balancing evaluation with critical thinking. An important part of any citizen's role is to endorse the actions of his or her government, but this must also be balanced by the citizen's willingness to criticize when that is called for.

---

[40] Allan Bloom, *The Closing of the American Mind* (New York: Touchstone, 1986), p. 230, 313–314.

Bloom was especially attracted to the activities of Socrates and his challenges to the Athenians, which finally resulted in the philosopher's death. The emphasis on community in the learning experience was vital to him even when it was unwelcome. I am reminded of the second grader, assigned a report on Socrates, who wrote, "Socrates lived in Athens, he talked a lot and they killed him." I have decided to be brief here.

Main Street, Wall Street, No Harm Street: Inseparable

A street is an indispensable, planned, designed, constructed passage to a destination hopefully beneficial to the well-being and functioning of the community. Sometimes they are dead ends, detours, one-way avenues, poorly maintained passageways, or roads of no return.

> To keep things in perspective, the ineluctable connection between our streets is spelled out succinctly by Laura Meckler in the *Wall Street Journal*. And as you read her projection, keep in mind an important given: follow the money.
>
> Is all this talk of the "fiscal cliff" making you sick? Actually, it's the other way around: The biggest long-term driver of the federal budget and its eye-popping deficit is health care. . . . All together, nearly one in four federal dollars is devoured by health-care spending. That is more than double the 10% of the budget it consumed in 1960, before Medicare and Medicaid were created. The Congressional Budget Office projects that in just a decade, health care will consume nearly one in three federal dollars, pressuring government spending.[41]

---

41 Laura Meckler, "Beneath Budget Battle, a Health-Spending Juggernaut," *Wall Street Journal*, December 18, 2012.

This medical superhighway is dominating the economy. We need to find more innovative, effective ways to keep us well and prevent our falling prey to bacteria and viruses that threaten our GDP just as they threaten us. It is more than justified since it represents not merely our comfort zones but life and death.

Chapter Seventeen

Perils of the Patient

Perils of the patient as victim mean that destructive medical/surgical experiences need to be verified. Well-intentioned defenders of patients' security and well-being often provide commonsense instruction on how to navigate the bewildering medical labyrinth for safe and effective treatment in the complex hospital arena. For example, surgical patients are advised to cancel a procedure if they are delayed beyond a given hour, such as 3:00 p.m., since this is presumed to frequently result in less favorable outcomes. Patients should request that doctors and nurses wash their hands; they should challenge the accuracy of a medical dosage; they should enquire whether their doctors are permitting interns to perform complex procedures, and so on. Some of these issues you will recall my addressing in detail since they are very important and have been given broad media coverage and support.

Doctor, wash your hands. Requesting that a doctor wash his or her hands if it appears that has not yet been done to stave off infection is crucial. World Health Organization (WHO) studies indicate that infection is the number-one killer in hospitals and in most cases is preventable. Commonsense suggestions are hygienically correct.

Hospital, regulate thyself. The medical institution should be accountable for the behavior of its own professionals and do whatever is necessary to supervise and regulate service standards. Many professionals are saying that historically the institutions have not done that very well. An assertive patient may find the blowback unexpected and intimidating, finally resulting in less effective treatment. For the patient, taking on the role of protagonist, being presumptive and pervasive, may unwittingly elicit antagonists in the medical community whose good will the patient desperately needs. That should not be the patient's role since it is doubtful most of us could do it well. As you may recall, I have confessed my own inadequacies in this regard. My recommendation for such well-meaning critics in the medical community is to accept their responsibility. Take up the orphaned boldness and adopt the challenge being foisted on the patient.

CNN's prime-time television presentation, "The Empowered Patient," covered twenty-five serious medical errors and irregularities. On most occasions they put the responsibility for protecting and correcting squarely on the back of the one least capable of intervening—the patient. The list includes babies stolen from the hospital, fake doctors, treating the wrong patient, pharmacy mix-ups, patients with the same last names, botched plastic surgery, dosage errors, and errors in discharge. The patient needs an advocate while being incapable of intervening personally. The patient may be medicated and unaware of the circumstances occurring, or may be personally reticent when facing those with the stature accorded medical professionals.

As journalist Elizabeth Cohen has put it: "No good doctor ever means to hurt you. Doctors and nurses and everyone who takes care of us are just like us, human and make mistakes. Now you can help them get things right."[42]

---

[42] Elizabeth Cohen, "25 Shocking Medical Mistakes," *CNN, aired June 9, 2012.*

The need for enforceable standards and medical regulations has been neglected, and an attempt has been made to impose this important responsibility on the least influential, who should be protected and should receive assured quality care as an institutional guarantee, rather than needing to personally police the job performance of medical professionals. It is another stark example of the systemic abandonment of accountability. This has resulted in part in the staggering casualty and death rate among patients. Several attempts at enforcing quality care have been attempted by groups advocating a patient's bill of rights, but they have met with very limited success. You could be the next compromised patient. So, let's look at where they do it, how they do it, why they do it, and how to change it!

Blowback may be the unfortunate result when patients seek to protect themselves. Such recommendations may be based on credible sources, but the patient's treatment and future at that institution with those medical professionals may be jeopardized by doing the "right" thing. On such occasions, though the patient is technically right, strategically he or she may be alienating the very people responsible for his or her welfare (life or death). The expected level of patient obsequiousness has not been met, and this is offensive to the system. I have made that mistake several times. It can be construed as arrogance and completely misunderstood. It is dangerous. Understand up front that the hospital is arguably the most hazardous institution in the world.

I have seen numerous recommendations for this misadventure in the media, TV, newspapers, and self-help magazines, urging patients to be their own arbiters, to take the bull by the horns and challenge any and all medical professionals. Our goal is to effectively influence the overall outcome for the good of the patient. But my experience has prompted a cautionary note to such advice, even though it is well intended. The medical professionals are the authority figures in their respective institutions, and the patient has not yet risen to the dignity of a coveted customer who can make that difference.

Drastically reduced future opportunities for attaining the service of outstanding surgeons and medical professionals befall the injured patient, adding insult to injury. Those medical specialists most capable of helping to restore health may be less accessible or even unavailable. Inflicted harm stigmatizes. The patient is compromised. A litany of medical complications inflicted through surgical injuries become as disqualifying as preexisting conditions prior to the Affordable Care Act.

Obtain, Read, and Study Your Medical Record

In order to be precise for interested patients and professionals, I will quote (and sum up from time to time) my own personal medical record. I urge all patients to obtain copies of their complete medical files, including doctor's notes. Once you have done this, you should read them carefully and become well informed. Your life depends on it. Discuss them with your doctors and question what you do not understand. For technical terms you may look to Google for definitions, pronunciations, and images, if so inclined. It's your body, and your life depends on how it is maintained. No one cares more than you!

Patient/Customer Expectations

Few other services are as blatantly and dangerously skewed toward the system's protection at the expense and detriment of the customer.

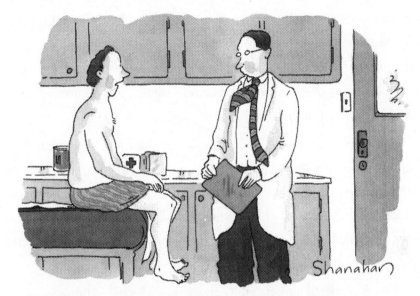

"And would you be performing the actual surgery?"

The vetting of a medical professional to perform a service is at times thwarted by the reluctance of the profession to practice quality control within their own ranks. As you might discover, perhaps surprisingly and painfully, an inexperienced and often incompetent intern might actually perform a surgery surreptitiously while you are expecting and deserving a highly skilled, experienced professional. If a student is nervously and tentatively learning at the patient's expense and jeopardy, unfortunately what is really learned may be unhelpful for all concerned. This recurrent arrangement has been discretely shrouded from you and me. The practice, you may be surprised to know, is one which medical professionals seldom tolerate with regard to themselves and their own families. It is an unacceptable double standard about life, death, fairness, and equality in providing medical service.

As mentioned previously, Dr. Atul Gawande is a renowned surgeon and author, and a member of the Harvard Medical School faculty. He recounted an atypical discussion with a fellow professional on this very sensitive subject. Noticing a picture of a colleague's adorable baby on his desk as they talked, he inquired if an intern had delivered the child. After an unpleasant pause, he was informed interns were not even allowed in the room!

Dr. Gawande expanded on the fairness issue as he related an incident involving his own infant son, a child with special needs. At just eleven days old, the child was diagnosed with a severe cardiac defect in which the aorta had not developed properly. Receiving that news challenged his own thinking and his position on this serious but little explored medical concern.

This is an arrow aimed at the conscience, a heartrending test of the principle versus the practice of medical fairness, with his own son's life and health at stake. Reading his account helped me realize how very difficult it would be to implement medical fairness—medical democracy—if doctors were in complete charge of the decision making. In this case, the situation was no longer an academic or philosophical consideration but a potential life-and-death issue for his own child. That can quite often be the case whenever a scheduled procedure is arranged. While Dr. Gawande's case was highly unusual, requiring a specialist's attention, the subject of fairness is the crux of the issue. What are the patient's rights? Are patients at greater risk than medical professionals since, for professionals, special treatment is routine? The issue is one of equality and fairness as life and death are in the balance.

When such risks are shared equally by all, experience indicates we will have better outcomes than we would if the risk can be evaded consistently by a select group. Medical treatment should not be arranged based on first-, second-, and third-class criteria. Medical democracy is our goal.

In the particular case above, a dedicated intern put in extended hours and effort on Dr. Gowanda's behalf and hoped to play a major role in further treatment for his son. He was displaced, however, as a highly qualified specialist was summoned, thus precluding routine support for the traditional model. Dr. Gawande went with the optimal choice, whom he knew had the superior vital experience and earned reputation. The personal illustration chosen to make his point reflects a very demanding situation, one that is not at all routine. I am not being critical of the doctor. I admire him. A question I have as I write this, though, is if an intern is not the best available source on critical medical decisions such as those illustrated here, shouldn't we all expect a qualified specialist to be obtained? That is fair. Love that democracy!

Several medical authors I consulted with while writing this book noted repeatedly how they made life-and-death decisions with very limited information and skills early in their careers, hence the validity of the "burying your mistakes" attitude. Dr. Gawande's use of his own son as an example is testimony to his commitment to fairness and honesty and helps us realize how we must all be protected by the system regardless of our social status or professional connections. It demonstrates how we must struggle with fairness to make this happen—and how very difficult it may be. In fact, this may point to another weakness in the system that should serve all equally regardless of social class when life-or-death issues are in play.

This also indicates why the medical system cannot regulate itself in many such dilemmas. Thus it is an obvious conclusion that on such vital matters, the system must initiate changes to function with fairness and equality. Choices about life and death and dispensing privilege must be established uniformly, even when—*especially* when—this is incredibly hard to facilitate because of what is at stake. Democracy, requiring equal opportunity, is seldom easy but is essential to our fundamental commitment as a society. Given the extreme example, few would fault the doctor's judgment. The issue, however, is a real one, and a double standard is not acceptable. The Golden Rule premise will help remind us what we do not yet have, except perhaps in the form of a lofty ideal. I quote the justification or rationalization of Dr. Gawande's sobering conclusion on this agonizing issue:

> The advantage of this coldhearted machinery is not merely that it gets the learning done. If learning is necessary but causes harm, then above all it ought to apply to everyone alike. Given a choice, people wriggle out, and those choices are not offered equally. They belong to the connected and the knowledgeable, to insiders over outsiders, to the doctor's child but not the truck driver's. If choice cannot go to everyone, maybe it is better when it is not allowed at all.[43]

The good doctor's last statement shows that he has a bold vision of humanitarian medical practice. He cautions that we need to face the reality of our limitations as we strive to overcome them rather than comfortably adapt. What I admire about him is that he doesn't duck the hard stuff.

---

[43] Gawande, *Complications*, pp. 32–33.

Elizabeth Warren, currently a first-term senator from Massachusetts, has been pushing legislation that will bring about fairer treatment for all in financial regulation. This is where Wall Street, Main Street, and No-Harm Street significantly influence one another.

Gretchen Morgenson talked with Senator Warren recently and shared this: "I interviewed her about her new memoir, A Fighting Chance, in which she discusses one of America's biggest challenges: how to level the playing field so that Main Street doesn't always come second to Wall Street."

The senator explained how her advisor, Lawrence H. Summers offered her solid information about how to situate herself in an upcoming election.

For those who may be unaware, I will list a few of Larry Summers's accomplishments: He was a recent president of Harvard University and secretary of the Treasury during the Clinton administration. He is the new chair of the board of directors at the Center for Global Development. Without a doubt, he is one of the most influential financial power brokers in the world. His counsel is priceless.

> "After dinner, Larry leaned back in his chair and offered me some advice," Ms. Warren writes. "I had a choice. I could be an insider or I could be an outsider. Outsiders can say whatever they want. But people on the inside don't listen to them. Insiders, however, get lots of access and a chance to push their ideas. People—powerful people—listen to what they have to say. But insiders also understand one unbreakable rule: *They don't criticize other insiders.*"
>
> While Ms. Warren contends that the deck in Washington is stacked against Main Street, she says she remains hopeful about working to level the playing field.[44]

---

[44] Gretchen Morgenson, "From Outside or Inside, the Deck Looks Stacked," *New York Times*, April 26, 2014.

One statement of fact for the senator and for you and me is vital for understanding how democracy is threatened by Big Money: "Insiders also understand one unbreakable rule: *They don't criticize other insiders*." Obviously this is a tantalizing proposition for many in public office. It may be the biggest money card in the game. Where does that kind of government leave the average citizen? "Of the people, by the people, for the people" will become a faint echo of our nations past greatness.

They are not only insiders; they are untouchable. That is not consistent with the fundamentals of democracy. You still have a vote; cherish it by using it wisely while you still have it. Whether it is regarding capitalism, commerce, or cures, our vote is our power.

Tribute to Our "Outsider" Truckers

I could not easily overlook the selection of the truck driver as a symbol, by Dr. Gawande, for the outsiders in the previous illustration, representing the class factor of those less likely to receive favorable medical treatment. The truckers, as depicted here, can't hope to control the quality and competency of the surgeons who may determine their families' medical outcomes. They may be randomly assigned a beginner without ever knowing it, even if their life hangs precariously in the balance. The good doctor does introduce an "ought" into the dilemma, perhaps hoping a mysterious magic wand of equality will somehow prevail. I remain convinced that if doctors were forced to endure incompetent interns treating their own loved ones as regularly as the rest of us, the system would soon change dramatically for the better! But without transparency, we cannot hope to trust that they will follow through with this very difficult practice.

The clear yet unsurprising breech of the moral dilemma—this inequality—is not about what car one drives, the size or location of a residence, one's zip code, the schools attended, or one's profession (except of course that doctors are automatically insiders by profession). This is about life and death and should be understood as such. Your life, as a patient in a democratic society, and the lives of your children, are as valuable as those of the doctors who are treating you or the members of your family. That is what democracy is about. When it comes to the quality of care they may expect, others are judged as unequal compared to doctors in the medical arena. And of course most of us knew that, but we may not have understood the full implications of our less-favorable class. Patients are regarded in this way (or should I say disregarded?) tacitly by the medical community. The doctors are depicted as connected, meaning their power over our lives may be elevated unfairly when they so choose. I have, during five surgeries and lengthy hospital stays, met some to whom I choose not to surrender that decision.

Don't Like to Think About It

The "average person" depicted symbolically, just as the truck driver, is labeled, categorized classified, and tucked crudely into a remote social stratum. These folks presumably do not merit life's full measure of equal opportunities because of what they do for their daily bread. They are depicted and depreciated because of their employment and presumed persona. You may have been wishing, as I have, that your life would be equally valued on that ultra index. There is more than a hint here that in the medical system it definitely is not, and there is little accountability over the delivery of services to justify—and implement—corrections for such inequalities. That is why we must hear loud and clear the patients' point of view.

We are talking about real people in a society oriented toward democratic equality who must be as highly valued as the head of the American Medical Association. That is our esteemed goal. See it clearly in your mind's eye as we strive to achieve it. We then move a bit closer to becoming what should by virtue of our values and rights in a community demonstrate our commitment to portray that city on a hill. The symbolic elevation and architecture won't compensate for our designated inequality. We have chosen, ideally, a medical democracy; nothing less will do and we should accept no less. We cannot countenance a national democracy with a medical aristocracy—the two are irreconcilable. That is not who we are.

The risks of any procedure must be clearly explained, including the principal surgeon's commitment to perform it. They should not delegate to an intern for educational or other purposes, without the patient's advanced consent. Level the medical playing field. Welcome to democracy—and to better medicine for all.

Don't Know and Can't Ask

In my daily reading, I frequently encounter accounts of horrific incidents of inept medical practice by those who should, given their inadequate skills, be ineligible to treat patients. Recently another sobering description of an intern brutalizing a patient made me recall the numerous experiences I encountered personally. Lest some think I have exaggerated our predicament, here is one more disclosure of an incident that should not have occurred. Dr. Pauline Chen shares this personal experience:

One night early in my internship, I received a frantic page for help from a fellow intern.

Seasoned nurses had been unable to draw a patient's blood, which senior doctors had ordered be done if his fever spiked, so they'd called the covering doctor, the first-year resident on call. For more than an hour he had poked at the patient's arms and legs, littering the floor with blood-stained gauzes, used alcohol swabs and crumpled syringe and needle packaging.

When the patient finally kicked him out of the room, howling, "I'll hit you if you come near me again!" he called the only people he thought he could: the other interns.

"We didn't have to draw blood in medical school," he confessed, his eyes red behind his Harry Potter spectacles. "My med school didn't think it was important for us to learn."

One of us did manage to get the required blood, but for the rest of the week, we were haunted by the feeling that any one of us could easily have been in the same situation.[45]

Notice that the empathy expressed here is for the incompetent intern. I, as a former patient, had a decidedly different reaction. I wanted to console the brutalized patient who had every reason to expect quality care only to be subjected to this trauma. What is this about "First do no harm?" Both the hospital administration and the physicians should have been summoned to accept responsibility for this medical debacle. The remainder of the article showed little encouragement toward significant improvement any time soon. There was the subtle caution that it is worse if you must have treatment during the summer, when you might experience the ominous "July Effect." That refers to an ongoing study indicating that most interns begin at hospitals during the summer months with little or no skill. Extensive medical research indicates that the mortality rate is

---

[45]   Pauline Chen, "Are Med School Grads Prepared to Practice Medicine?" *New York Times*, April 24, 2014.

significantly higher at that time. The euphemism, the July Effect, has made its way into the literature.

Medically Relevant Discrimination

Our society should not discount the importance of the equality-inequality continuum as it relates to financial and social mobility attrition among the middle and lower classes. In the past few decades, a diminishing middle class, determined by an eroding financial base, has drawn the attention of both political and economic participants. The relationship between this wealth and privilege inequity and its inherent negative social consequences is accelerating, and the impact is universally destructive.[46]

Lest this assessment appear inflated, I refer to a recent article published by a local newspaper, which showed that terminal cancer and poverty were clearly linked, as stated above; data were cited to support the researchers' conclusions.

Poverty is a key factor, and it has a moral connotation. People's deprivation of access to the basic human necessities cannot be defended in our culture, regardless of our ideological orientation. When people are suffering, we must do what is needed to meet their needs. A recent report underscores this reality. Sensitive persons need to sharpen their concern if they care about others who live a skip and a hop down the road.

Dr. Thomas George, an oncologist at Shands at the University of Florida, agreed.

---

[46] Richard Wilkinson and Kate Pickett, *The Spirit Level: Why Greater Equality Makes Societies Stronger* (New York, Bloomsbury Press, 2009), p. 263.

"What we're seeing in Florida is a magnification of what we're seeing in the rest of the country," he said. Or, at least, the Deep South.

"North Florida is really part of the Deep South. When you look across the Deep South, you find higher rates of just about everything," said Dr. Barbara Curbow, professor and chair of the Department of Behavioral Science and Community Health in the College of Public Health and Health Professions at UF.

"In this at-risk region, poverty and income inequalities are endemic. U.S. Census Bureau data from 2010 show that the northern part of the state (including the Panhandle, which the cancer report excludes) has the second-highest level of income inequality in the U.S., second only to Louisiana.

The cancer report found 21 percent of the population in the North Florida region lives below the poverty line.

In Alachua County, for example, there are 730 patients for every primary care physician. In Union, that jumps to 5,184 patients per physician.

A dearth of doctors is part of the problem; but other factors contribute to the lack of access to health care. The recent cancer report found that 28 percent of people in Alachua County don't have insurance, so they just don't go to the doctor.

In Alachua County, 71 percent of women reported getting mammograms, compared with just 51 percent in Union County.[47]

As inequality continues to increase, with devastating consequences, a distinguished publication has challenged the hallowed economic trickle-down philosophy, and its relevance in a democratic society is dramatic. A French economist, Thomas Piketty, has swept into economic celebrity by taking on the oligarchic trend currently imposed by recent Supreme Court decisions—Money is Speech; Corporations are People; *Citizens United*—allowing unlimited and untraceable money to flow into the democratic process,

---

[47]   Kristine Crane, "Rural Areas Drive Region's High Cancer Death Rates," *Gainesville Sun*, March 24, 2013.

thus buying access and influence under the guise of free speech. Piketty argues convincingly that this is opposed to "one person, one vote" democratic systems. The very wealthy are outnumbered in a system such as ours and are making bold maneuvers at the highest level to bring this democratic structure under their firm control. For one such as Piketty to emerge on the scene with such stature, with impeccable scholarly credentials, in a heated electoral climate, is rare.

Steven Erlanger, of the *New York Times*, interviewed Mr. Piketty recently and came away with these observations:

> "So inequality has been quickly gathering pace, aided to some degree by the Reagan and Thatcher doctrines of tax cuts for the wealthy. Trickle-down economics could have been true," Mr. Piketty said simply. "It just happened to be wrong...."
>
> "In 2012 the top 1 percent of American households collected 22.5 percent of the nation's income, the highest total since 1928. The richest 10 percent of Americans now take a larger slice of the pie than in 1913, at the close of the Gilded Age, owning more than 70 percent of the nation's wealth. And half of that is owned by the top 1 percent."
>
> But he accepts that his work is essentially political, and he is highly critical of the huge management salaries now in vogue, saying that "the idea that you need people making 10 million in compensation to work is pure ideology."
>
> But like the Columbia University economist Joseph E. Stiglitz, he argues that extreme inequality "threatens our democratic institutions." Democracy is not just one citizen, one vote, but a promise of equal opportunity."[48]

---

[48]   Steven Erlanger, "Taking on Adam Smith (and Karl Marx)," *New York Times*, April 19, 2014.

To Presume Medical Democracy

I advocate this advance in our medical (democratic) equality, fully realizing that it may sound Pollyannaish, however sorely needed. We will risk that criticism coming from those who would contend that nothing should ever be done for the first time.

Certain concepts or cultural positions appear alien (not in a negative sense but unthinkable to the degree that implementation seems light-years away). We must bulk up the muscles of our mind. We must first think it, before we can develop and embellish it. It is unthinkable only because we have not yet challenged ourselves to consider it. We must conceptualize and share it with those we trust so they will not dismiss us as foolish.

Democracy alone is like that for the uninitiated and medical democracy even more so. To fashion equality of medical rights when we are mulling over India's richest man, America's top ten billionaires, and so on, sounds untouchable. It is only as we begin to talk about it, think about it, visualize it, that we can begin to evolve. It must be created, then from that flicker or spark it will progress. Otherwise, one may say we are talking nonsense, meaning no shared sense. Medical democracy in a functioning democracy will be one day more alien by its absence. It makes incredibly good sense, medically, as we will demonstrate later. It is important that we do this now, at a time when our cultural mobility is no longer upward but downward. Medical equality is much more humane. We cannot arrive at our destination without undertaking that journey.

The plan for medical equality has significant implications for the administration of justice and fairness in our major institutional delivery systems. Several sources have attributed 90 percent of the wealth of our nation to the top 1 percent of our population, and it may now be even more polarized. This represents a dramatic redeployment toward a cultural, financial and social inequality. This is inseparable from our medical participation with the severe social and moral implications that service encompasses.

Medical Madness

Chapter Eighteen

Applied Medical Mythology

Not all gods were Greeks; some were hatched in med school from ethereal eggs. How some doctors and surgeons view themselves compared with their peers and patients is of interest here because of the behavioral predictability it signifies. They now appear suspended precariously on a bungee cord of medical mythology, characterizing the professionals and profession, with an aura of veneration no longer accepted or relevant, and in modern society, bordering on the preposterous.

Some in the profession appear to have been foisted upon an awestruck public with the indication that they possessed nearly superhuman intelligence, superb performance skills, endurance, and brilliance, corresponding to infallibility and meriting total trustworthiness. The following example, offered by Dr. Paul Ruggieri in his autobiography, *Confessions of a Surgeon*, is revealing because it comes from a doctor's own published exposé. He shares some of his early perceptions as he entered this field of service. His book then depicts important behavioral corollaries—not all commendable. As we shall see, what one believes may make a difference.

Doctors or Deities?

A biography can excavate kernels of truth in a way that may seldom surface otherwise. There exists a presumed commitment to full disclosure, based on a presumption of a measure of immunity from moral responsibility for consequences, similar to that disclosed in the ritual of a religious confessional. Here I quote the good doctor's autobiography:

> I could see that surgeons were independent thinkers, relying only on themselves for success. Surgeons were gods. They also appeared to make a lot of money. I wanted to be a surgeon. . . . I was in awe of the surgical residents' stamina and ability to function on very little sleep. . . . It was twenty-four hours on and twenty-four hours off in the emergency room for six weeks. . . . I dared not ask for help in evaluating someone; it would have been considered a sign of weakness. It was never a spoken rule, but showing weakness of any kind was out of the question. It wasn't an option. Everyone who wanted to advance understood it.[49]

Their medical deity is dead. This irrationality has become a casualty of transparency. The curious, archaic mythical creature of the past must go the way of other mythologies that have long outlived their usefulness. The notion of patient insignificance and abject ignorance is obsolete. The new mantra must be "by patients, for patients," which can resonate as a contribution long overdue in supporting the inevitable coming systemic changes from without and within.

Feet of Clay

Encouraging mortals to assume the attributes of gods will expose in hindsight a most unfortunate medical failing with far-reaching negative side effects. Most, in the final analysis, will be proven to have feet of clay. Operating with very little sleep, constrained by

---

[49]   Ruggieri, pp. 8–10.

fatigue, bound by unspoken pretenses of omniscience, doctors put patients' lives at risk and the psyches of physicians in question. Most everyone outside the medical profession and hopefully on the inside, despite the apparent attempt by some at brainwashing, really knows that. A medical culture endorsing doctors' presumed infallibility, not permitting them to expunge ignorance with enlightenment as the situation demands, thus repeatedly jeopardizing patients, is beyond foolish. It is despicable. A mythical medical culture that behaves in ways that put our lives in danger is immoral and irrational. Maybe a four-letter word is called for: sick. Small wonder they have developed a reputation for burying their mistakes, the deification of the doctor notwithstanding. Killing the living to preserve an unspeakable code of honor is hardly a virtue and is in fact itself in urgent need of a somber requiem and burial.

Allow me to share one more revealing and sobering episode from Dr. Ruggieri's disclosures as he embraces his philosophy of medicine:

> I laughed as I cut another hole in Jane's intestine. "Why are you laughing, Paul?" Dr. Jenkins was puzzled. I laughed because it took less energy than crying. "Erin, I trained in a totally different era and I am not that old. There was never a limit on the number of hours I could work. There was never a clock to punch. On the contrary, it was a sign of strength to stay up as long as possible. Sure, after about a hundred hours, everything was a blur, but it was a character-building blur. It may not have been good for my patients then, but it is good for them now."[50]

This concise narrative is a brief segment of a dialogue that took place at 3:00 a.m. as Dr. Ruggieri, the general surgeon, responded to an on-call summons. He needed to remove adhesions from the

---

[50] Ruggieri, pp. 234–235.

patient of a surgical gynecologist who had found the patient's ovaries encased by the adhesions, which laced around the intestines and thus blocked the path of the gynecologist, preventing her from completing her planned surgical procedure.

A Character-Building Blur?

The surgeon recounts how he accidentally cut a half dozen holes in the patient's intestine, requiring sutures, as he clumsily extracted the adhesions to prepare for the planned original surgery. One puzzling comment I must repeat: "It may not have been good for my patients then, but it is good for them now." In other words, he has the audacity to say that his recounted historical experience was good for present patients as he mutilated the intestines of the patient he was called upon to assist! It was a learning experience. What is important here is the account of this sobering visit to the OR and noting the risk incurred by the patient in this horrific incident involving the dead-tired, belligerent, and bizarre general surgeon.

Transparency was desperately needed there. The medical community often vigorously denies fatigue's debilitating effects, which we will address later. How much permanent damage was inflicted? Did the patient survive? If so, was the patient ever told of the harm she suffered at his hands? Why didn't the other surgeon put a stop to the surgery? These necessary questions speak volumes about the lack of accountability in our system. The account also raises serious questions about the surgeon's touted "character-building" training noted in his rambling monologue. What has this to do with character?,And how many innocent casualties are required? How many mistakes did he bury from those appalling learning experiences? What he has shown us in this snapshot does not speak well for the education and practice that produced it.

Dr. Pauline Chen relates the difficulty the medical community is having in reforming its appalling practice of performing as though its members were not subject to the physiological limits affecting the remainder of the human race. We refer your attention to a few choice quotes from her *New York Times* article:[51]

> Over the past decade, in response to public concerns about medical errors arising from fatigue, the Accreditation Council for Graduate Medical Education, the organization responsible for accrediting American medical residency programs, has been progressively limiting the number of hours that trainees can work. . . .
>
> The latest mandate, which took effect in 2011, is the most stringent and deals most specifically with interns. These youngest doctors are allowed to work no longer than 16 hours in a day; and residency programs that violate the restriction risk losing their accreditation.
>
> The problem? Trying to do the same amount of work in fewer hours. . . .

The narrative becomes more confusing as the medical authorities attempt to clarify. Overwork and fatigue are juxtaposed, with the former being deemed more debilitating. Many laypersons would likely see these concepts as interrelated and contributing to the danger of performing hospital services poorly.

> "Fatigue is bad, but overwork is worse," said Dr. Lara Goitein, lead author of a recently published editorial in JAMA Internal Medicine and a pulmonary and critical care physician at Christus St. Vincent Regional Medical Center in Santa Fe, N.M. . . .

---

[51]   Pauline W. Chen, M.D. "The Impossible Workload for Doctors in Training, Fatigue and Consequences—Kill Patients," New York Times, April 18, 2013.

"It's as if you told airline pilots that they could only work a certain number of hours, but they had to fly 50 percent more flights," Dr. Goitein said. . . .

"You can't keep asking these young doctors to do more and more work in less time without affecting patient care," Dr. Goitein said. "Until we address the problem of overwork, we're just playing a shell game."

Overwork and fatigue are to me clearly linked, if not indistinguishable or closely related issues. Find overwork and expect fatigue to be nearby. Attempting to separate them obfuscates the problem and creates additional dilemmas for strategies of improvement.

I doubt seriously if you wish to have an overly tired surgeon, whether intern or seasoned professional, wielding a life-altering scalpel or risking your life with a potentially lethal prescription that, if not administered with precision, can also kill. Rushing to perform more in less time makes no sense whatsoever as an intended solution for the conundrum of patient safety resulting from fatigue. There is more here than correlation; causation should be expected. I really have difficulty understanding why fatigue would not be assumed as a result of overwork. As a layman, I can only generalize, but this appears to give the impression of a disguise. The problem is very serious. Well-chosen words are the best avenue between inquiring minds. They may then know how to accomplish mutual goals.

As described in a 2010 article in the *Wall Street Journal*, new guidelines from the Accreditation Council for Graduate Medical Education would limit the number of hours and suggest increased supervision for medical residents.

Amid continued concern about errors by overworked medical residents, hospitals would be forced to curtail shifts and increase supervision of some doctors-in-training under proposed new guidelines for residency programs released Wednesday. . . . These worries led the Accreditation Council for Graduate Medical Education, ACGME, in 2003 to limit resident hours to 80 hours a week. Until then, some were regularly working up to 120 hours a week, according to the council.[52]

A doctor accumulating 120 hours per week, would log over seventeen hours per day for seven days. I would most assuredly bypass the services of that professional if I had any information about his or her horrendous schedule.

In an article in the *Harvard University Gazette*, Dr. William J. Cromie, renowned staff researcher, states that not only are residents overworked, but they are also subject to guilt and subsequent loss of empathy:

What is more, most of the interns (83.6 percent) reported that, even in the year after the standards were introduced, they worked more hours than allowed. And the Harvard study shows that things have not gotten any better. "Even interns who worked less than the current limits, but who continued to work five to nine extended-duration shifts per month, had eight times greater odds of reporting preventable medical errors that harmed patients," Czeisler says. "These errors included more than four times [4.6] more fatalities than those committed by interns who did not work extended shifts."[53]

---

[52] Shirley S. Wang, "New Rx for Young Doctors: Shorter Work Day," *Wall Street Journal*, June 24, 2010.

[53] William J. Cromie, "Doctor Fatigue Hurting Patients: Interns Feel Guilt, Lose Empathy," *Harvard University Gazette*, December 14, 2006.

Insiders Are the Deciders

Inequality in medical treatment is depicted as a presumptive factor in the mutilation of the intestines by the overly tired surgeon attacking adhesions. We do not wish to assume the medical community is immune to the debilitating impact of fatigue on their performance.

Experience has demonstrated that the risks of fatigue are especially acute in professions like health care, as well as among airline pilots and air traffic controllers, and in truck driving and manufacturing, which all involve overnight shifts where careless errors can endanger lives. Truckers have learned a bit about the dangers of operating a potentially lethal vehicle when overly tired. They have developed an array of regulations protecting them and us, and these are closely enforced. Might I add here that even as "outsiders," they may have one up on some in the medical profession, who seem to have been indoctrinated differently by their mentors. The potentially lethal effects of fatigue, when stretched beyond determined limits, have been disregarded by the profession—with disastrous consequences.

The casualties from medical errors are abundant and have been ignored far too long. Too many believe in the cult of a mythical superior endurance that is an exception to normal human limitations; this is supposed to come with being a doctor. Sorry, but those who posture as gods and goddesses are mere mortals in denial. They are more like you and me than they care to admit, except for their misplaced belief in their own propaganda and their operation under the influence of their own rapidly vanishing halos. Our truckers appear at least to know some of their human limitations and, as a group, may be setting a better example than some in the medical profession.

For instance, the US Department of Transportation and the Federal Motor Carrier Safety Administration have very strict "hours of service" rules, which, while not perfect, do protect us from the independent and occasionally reckless abandon we have witnessed routinely in the medical profession's apparent disregard for the debilitating effects of fatigue. Calling attention to the truckers and contrasting their fatigue-related regulations with those of the medical community is revealing. As our "do no harm" edict presumes, fatigue should be diligently addressed, given its demonstrated effect on "complications." As insiders and deciders, medical personnel should take appropriate action to protect the patient from harm. Sweeping regulations will be necessary. Their clamor to maintain self-regulation will be fierce even as their representatives confess that the hospital is the world's most dangerous institution, killing nearly one hundred thousand per year through preventable medical errors. Many of the more obvious reasons for this carnage have been referenced above.

When burying your mistakes is a standard practice, it is absolutely abhorrent. We sincerely hope that transparency will project a screen of sanity for those in the profession who are too frequently strained, as indicated by the episodes cited in this book. It is sorely needed, from the patient's point of view, and we hope from that of the medical profession as well. As the nation turns its attention toward a noble goal of equitable treatment for all citizens, we have begun to realize the intensity of the fissure in which the profession has been practicing. Time to stop digging and start behaving as their medical manifesto professes they do.

Chapter Nineteen

Rationing Medical Treatment
Endangers All

Howard Hughes was right! The obsessive-compulsive aviator and scientist was ahead of the current medical profession when it came to understanding the danger of marauding microorganisms. Many will recall the dramatic scene in the movie *The Aviator* (directed by Martin Scorsese), in which Hughes was transfixed by that terrifying doorknob. As we struggle presently to sound the alarm in our hospitals and related health care facilities, installing video cameras, hiring hygiene police to corral detractors, we have hardly made a dent in reckless behavior. Infections from bacteria and viruses decimate our institutions, and we remain puzzled that we cannot martial the allegiance of the brightest and best among us to be eternally vigilant on the most important medical line of defense. Simple hand washing by all has proven most difficult to initiate and maintain—yet when practiced unfailingly, it is most effective.

We do not wish the burden of OCD on our professions; but let's face it, some eighty years ago Hughes was way ahead of us, even with his eccentric and at times paralyzing demeanor. He knew better than we did what could be lurking on that innocent-looking doorknob. Microorganisms are moving among us at our peril. An alert, informed, and hygienically sophisticated populace is an integral part of your and my personal health. The availability of needed services is a good defense. Given what we now know, that is simple common sense.

The nature of disease transmission and community protection or immunity appears to support the collective availability of medical services to all, independent of their personal financial resources. Think about this example: Dr. Jonas Salk discovered the inoculation formula to prevent the polio virus from ravaging the body and either crippling or killing its victim. That was the beginning of the end for the scourge of polio we had come to fear. The history is so well known that we will not elaborate on the details of its development. At the time the vaccine was developed, my family resided in a small college community of about four thousand. I recall vividly standing in line one summer afternoon excitedly chatting with others around us about the wonders of this great gift of medical science, the eradication of polio. But consider this hypothetical: Suppose we had taken the position that the vaccine should be deemed a commodity available only to those who could afford the market price of a dose—if not, too bad. The eradication of this terrible disease was dependent on all citizens becoming immune; we were all in this together as a society. The health of one was dependent on the health of all. That same logic is true of many medical applications. The remedy is collective health care, regardless of how that may wreak havoc with popular ideologies. The community's health is a community issue, and medical responsibility is equivalent to national defense.

A thrilling medical news bulletin recently carried this improbable message, celebrating the conquest of polio in India. What makes this even more exciting is that the conquest of this disease involves a nation that has poverty levels that dwarf any we have known in our worst recessions. According to the article in the *Wall Street Journal*:

> The World Health Organization plans to say on Monday that India has gone exactly three years since recording its last polio case, one of the biggest public-health achievements of recent times, and

one that could set the stage for stamping out the ancient scourge globally.

Public-health officials now hope to officially certify India as polio free in coming weeks.

Many long doubted that India could pull it off, given the country's size, poor sanitation and the enormous challenge of vaccinating millions of children, often in far-flung places and in the face of societal and religious resistance.

But stamping out an ancient and debilitating disease promises much more. "The benefits of eradication accrue for eternity," said Dr. Jafari of WHO.[54]

Tragically Neglected—Mental Health Services

My encounter with schizophrenia is a disturbing example resulting in part from rationed care in the mental health area and a fledgling attempt on my part at offering help when none was available. A very distraught parishioner whose son had intermittent bouts with schizophrenia approached me unexpectedly. They lacked resources for ongoing professional healthcare and treatment. For severe lapses, assistance had been available in a large city a substantial distance away. On this occasion, I was approached midmorning by his mother with the lament "My son believes he is Jesus! Can you help me?" I had no certified training to authorize my involvement in this situation. But we had always tried to be helpful with dysfunctional family issues, and I was available. This is an intense example of the variety of human perils I experienced in my work. Having taken graduate courses in abnormal psychology only made me more apprehensive. (Keep in mind, too, that this was in

---

[54] Gautam Naik and Nikita Lalwani, "India Manages to Free Itself of Polio: Against-Odds Achievement Remains Fragile but Brings Global Eradication Quest Tantalizingly Close," *Wall Street Journal*, January 12, 2014.

the early sixties; the science dictating treatments and attitudes has changed significantly.)

Within minutes the troubled mother, appearing terrified, entered my office with her son. He had a rather glazed and distant look. He was college age but not enrolled in school at the time. I picked up a Bible with the words of Jesus printed in red, addressed the young man as Jesus, and led him to a comfortable chair. I opened the Bible to the New Testament and noted that the verses indicated what he had said when he had been on Earth so long ago, and that he might be interested in reading it. To my relief, he took the Bible and began reading silently.

His mother in the meantime was attempting to make arrangements for a psychiatric analysis at the same institution that had treated him previously. I remained with him while she prearranged the appointment and transportation. That took over an hour, and I was reassured when she returned. The really delicate part then became whether he would consent to go. I was invited to accompany them and agreed, feeling it would be unhelpful if I declined. There were four of us in the car: "Jesus," his father, his mother, and me. I was even more nervous during the trip, realizing that at any moment he could exit the automobile and we would have virtually no means of getting him to voluntarily return.

In a few encounters with the father, I found him to be a brilliant man, given to periods of acute withdrawal. I was impressed with his grasp of current scientific theory despite his having had no advanced education; he was a high school dropout and was troubled by bouts of alcoholism. The son had appeared acutely introverted and withdrawn, so it was difficult to evaluate him in that regard.

I was impressed at that time with people who could display extraordinary memorization capabilities, having myself chosen to memorize every scheduled presentation I gave. For over ten years, I would laboriously yet meticulously commit each presentation to memory, including paragraph-length quotes from distinguished authors. I would challenge myself by keeping abreast of the time it took to master pages and perfect a single successful repetition. Regardless of the occasion (commencement addresses, university chapel services, etc.), I carried no notes to the podium. To my delight I found that I got substantially better with practice—tripling my performance in memorization. Just to dispel any extravagant pretense, I must point out that actors do this routinely, so it was no big deal!

His father knew about this peculiarity of mine and wished to share his own extraordinary talent in that regard. His memory really was a gift. On one occasion he handed me a book and invited me to open it anywhere and scan a few pages. Having done that, I handed it back and watched as he flipped through those same pages, and viewed each for less than a minute. He then handed the book back to me and proceeded, to my astonishment, to quote each page with remarkable accuracy. Even though his son was impaired so severely as to be virtually dysfunctional, this gentleman was quite intelligent and had an enviable gift for memorization.

Certain mental illnesses can be accompanied with remarkable and distinctive psychological attributes or tradeoffs. You may recall the book and film *A Beautiful Mind*, which portrayed the life of John Nash, a Nobel laureate in economics. Asperger's syndrome carries symptoms of severe interpersonal withdrawal that have resulted in pinpointed concentration allowing some to achieve mentally in ways that were beyond normal. These are of course the rare exceptions.

In writing this I am reminded that Einstein's son, Eduard, was schizophrenic. He had to be institutionalized and despite his apparent talent was unable to function socially. The treatments of that era, especially electroshock therapy, were devastating. Father and son had very little time together.[55]

We Are All in This Together

Horrible bacteria and viruses, from the flu virus to flesh-eating bacteria, and mental afflictions can become almost too terrible to contemplate. Again, the health of the community depends on citizens availing themselves of redeeming antidotes from existing medical resources.

The availability of service must be offered equally, regardless of the ability to pay, if that premise is to be initiated and fulfilled. That has certain implications for making nationally supported health care available for all equally—a nod to our medical democracy. When it comes to this, you can be selfish in your outlook or charitable, but the behavior is the same. It must be offered equally for the community to gain the strategic advantage and defeat these deadly microorganisms. Community security is also sacrificed when mental health is skirted. Regardless of how we may feel personally about someone who cannot pay for their medical coverage, the medical support must be available, or we risk the health of the entire community. Common sense, if not caring, must determine our judgment to assure service.

Viruses and bacteria are hoping we leave some straggling, unprotected victims for them to feast upon and thus enable them to

---

[55] Walter Isaacson, *Einstein: His Life and Universe* (New York: Simon & Schuster, 2007).

then spread to the rest of the population. This is a team sport, and we are all players. There are no spectators; health is everybody's game. We are not competing with other members of our society but with alien microorganisms. One cannot be too healthy in this contest. The bacteria and viruses continue their evasive maneuvers. Mutational changeovers persist to outwit us, as we are often lax in the 24/7 efforts required to maintain due vigilance. The virus we prepared for yesterday is not what we may meet today—and certainly not tomorrow.

Numerous countries are displaying an accelerating interest in combating a variety of diseases. Severe acute respiratory syndrome (SARS) in China resulted in several hundred deaths in Asia and Canada a decade ago. Ebola from Africa has reached pandemic dimensions there and is threatening us here. Lethal lung infections, called Middle East respiratory syndrome (MERS), journeys from Saudi Arabia. These are but the tip of the iceberg; action is needed and appears to be building momentum.

According to an editorial in the *New York Times*, "A five-year program to extend assistance to 30 countries to protect their populations could cost the United States up to $1.5 billion, which would be worth spending if the initial projects prove successful."[56]

An informative *Frontline* special, "Hunting the Nightmare Bacteria," aired on PBS on October 22, 2013, and awakened us to these deadly organisms for which we are frighteningly unprepared.[57] The discussion of Pfizer's role in this drama was the most instructive. Dr. Charles Knirsch, infectious disease specialist and the company's

---

[56] Editorial, "Coping with Infectious Disease," *New York Times*, February 21, 2014.

[57] Rick Young, producer. "Hunting the Nightmare Bacteria," *Frontline*. PBS, October 22, 2013.

vice president of clinical research, led Pfizer's side of the enlightening discussion, charting their dramatic retreat from the vital area of antibiotic research. Stay with my sports metaphor for a moment: In tennis I relished the opportunity of engaging a more gifted opponent for the contribution it made to my own game. That opponent would challenge me to raise the level of my performance and enhance my skills. I became a better player and was then able to compete at a higher level. It seems the bacterial world is a little like this, though their enhancing capacity in the face of human opposition is exponential compared to ours. They have been known to morph into world-class status, enhancing their ability to kill us in a matter of minutes.

Consider this exchange with Dr. Knirsch:

Dr. Knirsch: The bacteria have the advantage really is what it comes down to. Their doubling time is in a matter of minutes and hours, so the opportunity with every new organism that is dividing is the chance for a recombinational event or some way around the therapeutic that is designed to treat that bacteria. I think that even with appropriate use, you will see the emergence of resistance.

From idea to a medicine, it takes about 10 years when you succeed. . . .

Interviewer: So you decided essentially to shift the capital away from antibiotics and toward vaccine platforms.

Dr. Knirsch: Yes, Pfizer made a decision to move from antibiotics to vaccines even though they had a team of the most prestigious in the world at the time. The issue surrounded the need the company felt to best serve the shareholders. Prevention via vaccines appeared to tip the balance over cures and they have moved abruptly in that direction.

The discussion then proceeded to the role of government in support of these long-term issues. The implication being that the private sector was not as well equipped to pursue decades-long commitments with less than certain outcomes. The risk to the shareholder, given the nature of the market, was not conducive to it.

The conversation gravitated naturally to the role of capitalism for these projects. The issue of capitalism's failure, so to speak, was handled delicately by conceding that the National Institutes of Health was a great partner and sorely needed in this endeavor. The logic for abandoning antibiotics and moving resources to vaccines was defended by emphasizing their preventive nature and that, if they are effective, some of the need for antibiotics might be reduced. Both dimensions of the medical research were deemed necessary. For Pfizer, the decision centered upon market forces with a pronounced emphasis on government involvement to pick up vital components of long-term medical research. And so it must, regardless of how those with ideological differences may construe this movement. The life and health of our society and the world are dependent on maintaining accelerated programs to meet these needs.

The *Wall Street Journal* recently carried some exciting news. Several pharmaceutical companies are returning to the development of antibacterial medications. They were quite candid about profit being the key factor in their abandonment of that specific avenue of R&D.

It is broadly acknowledged that we are lagging behind while treacherous microorganisms have surged ahead. Window dressing regarding the difficulties in discovery and manufacture of these vital drugs is implicit. It still comes down to profit. With that understood, let's become selfish. The stockholders and directors have families who are just as vulnerable to these diseases as anyone else. This concerns their survival too. Let's propose a toast to our own survival! It is the killer bugs or us. Which will it be? Come on, folks—this is not a difficult decision. Greed will not prevent these lethal life forms from launching pandemic invasions. Our medical geniuses are among the brightest professionals on the planet. Get on with it, whatever it takes!

With the spread of superbugs, the importance of antibiotics has once again assumed a crucial role in the ongoing attempt to control international disease. Though drug companies have claimed that antibiotics aren't financially viable, some are beginning to rethink their research and development aims.

> Another Boston startup, Enbiotix, is in discussions with multiple big drug makers interested in a deal, including those without active anti-infectives divisions, according to its chief executive, Jeff Wager.
> "Antibiotics are never going to be huge blockbusters," Mr. Wager says. "And yet the short answer is, we need these drugs. I don't think big pharma can call themselves good corporate citizens without them."[58]

The *New York Times* recently commented on "The Rise of Antibiotic Resistance." In an article published May 10, 2014, the *Times* editorial board discussed the disturbing results of a World Health Organization report that shows antimicrobial resistance in bacteria, viruses, and parasites is increasing:

> A problem so serious that it threatens the achievements of modern medicine," the organization said. "A post-antibiotic era, in which

---

[58] Hester Plumridge, "Drug Makers Tiptoe Back into Antibiotic R&D: As Superbugs Spread, Regulators Begin to Remove Roadblocks for New Treatments" *Wall Street Journal*, January 23, 2014.

common infections and minor injuries can kill, far from being an apocalyptic fantasy, is instead a very real possibility for the 21st century."

The growth of antibiotic-resistant pathogens means that in ever more cases, standard treatments no longer work, infections are harder or impossible to control, the risk of spreading infections to others is increased, and illnesses and hospital stays are prolonged.[59]

It seems that almost every day, new information becomes available about the ability of resistant bacteria to take down a population. Again, these are organisms that don't discriminate on the basis of race, religion, or financial status.

---

[59] Editorial, "The Rise of Antibiotic Resistance," *New York Times*, May 10, 2014.

Chapter Twenty

System Failing Ailing Patients

Drastically reduced future opportunities for attaining the service of outstanding surgeons and medical professionals befall the medically injured patient, adding insult to injury. Those medical specialists most capable of helping to restore health may be less accessible or even completely unavailable. Inflicted harm stigmatizes, and the patient is compromised. Prior to the Affordable Care Act, a litany of medical complications inflicted through surgical injuries was as disqualifying as a preexisting condition. There should be a moral obligation from the medical profession to the patient to provide the best treatment, in addition to and beyond any purely economic issue (though it is an economic issue as well). Remember the primary goal is to serve the patient; the commitment is to their health. How then can patients countenance being treated as outsiders as a result of medical errors? Or have patients become accustomed to—and do they now even anticipate—such discriminatory behavior as natural, not to be questioned or challenged? It is accepted by assumption.

Patience of Patients

By assuming every advantage, the medical system has long demonstrated its dominance over patients when time, place, convenience, urgency, and secrecy are superimposed with little regard for the patient's wishes, needs, and well-being. When one embraces that mantle of authority, operated by and for those deemed to be superior (insiders, if you will), adjustment becomes a matter of convenience to amicably avoid conflict and confrontation. Going along with the demands temporarily reduces tension, but in most encounters the patients' needs are really secondary. That, too, must change if we are to improve this ailing and failing medical system.

Transparency and Accountability

We have heard a lot about transparency of late, and it will reappear several times further along in the book. It has become highly touted as a mechanism for improving our systems and institutions. Critical medical insiders and outsiders regard it as a means whereby the current medical system can begin to undergo positive change. The widespread use of the video camera, among other innovations, has been recommended as a verification instrument of choice for buttressing transparency and accountability.

"Believe Me or Your Lying Eyes?"

The absence of transparency in our present structure prevents us from allocating responsibility for procedures for which service providers could be held accountable for second-rate or negligent surgical or medical outcomes. Transparency's absence obfuscates performance outcomes and responsibility, and leads to corruption. While seeing is not always believing, it is a leg up on most other alternatives. As Groucho Marx famously asked, "Who are you going to believe, me or your lyin' eyes?"

Increased transparency as a standard would assure improved support for medical professionals performing at their best and learning from their experiences. Since they would be under constant surveillance for evaluation of performance, the option or reassurance of concealment would be gone. This would enhance the performance incentive of the competent and threaten to expose and at times depose the consistently incompetent. Patients would then be assured of more reliable and unbiased accountability by the institutions serving them. The cost of repetitive medical procedures, now borne mostly by the patient, would be more fairly allocated.

What the medical establishment could not do via its commitment to the patient, they would become compelled to do by virtue of the disclosing power of the camera. Now everybody knows! Profits, increasingly in the coffers of private equity investors, could and should be allocated for payment of damages to injured patients when warranted. Inferior incentives stemming from poorly monitored evaluative criteria in the business community would be regarded as a moral hazard. For medical practitioners, the stated intention to "do no harm" would become a more neutralizing euphemism confirmed by the institution's fairness.

Prophets on Profits

Systems attempting to function with profit as their primary purpose for existing are destined to fail. In the medical system, profit as the prime directive is a recipe for disaster. Profit must be the servant, not the master. I'm not arguing that money should be excluded from medicine, but it should be properly prioritized.

How Profit Discovered America

Our infant nation did not discover profit on this vast continent, endemic to the verdure of Jamestown, embedded in the soil. The first settlers brought the concept from Europe, which they had left needing to unburden and purify themselves from the constraints they felt had been imposed by an alien authority on that continent. Personal quests and vast opportunities as spacious as this new land spurred them on. As they saw it, God had provided them with a compass and the assurance that loyalty and obedience, as they understood them, would be the only condition for achievement.

In *An Empire of Wealth*, historian J. S. Gordon explains:

> New England was not founded by men bent first of all on adventure and profit. Instead, the most important reason for settling there was to build a city on a hill . . . unmolested by corruption, according to God's commandments.
>
> But that city, to be sure, is a project still under construction after nearly four hundred years. . . . Nor were the Puritans in the least averse to prosperity in this world as long as the worship of God came first. Indeed, they regarded it as a sign of God's grace, a sign that the individual was indeed saved. Sixteenth and seventeenth-century merchants, many of them, Puritans, would often write at the head of their ledgers, "In the name of God and profit."[60]

Rich Lowery, editor of the *National Review* and prominent political analyst, emphasizes how swiftly and thoroughly the Puritans made their memorable mark on this rugged and vibrant New World—new to them at least but inhabited by people whose lives and cultures they considered totally alien, primitive, barbaric, and of course inferior.

---

[60] J. S. Gordon, *An Empire of Wealth: The Epic History of American Economic Power* (New York: Harper Collins Publishers, 2004), p. 27.

He offers an assessment of their early encounters and accomplishments:

> The settlers who poured into New England included tradesmen of all sorts, bringing their hustle and shrewdness. They quickly resorted to technology to make up for the relative absence of labor. The first sawmill opened in 1634; a dozen were operating by 1650. John Winthrop's son took an interest in industry and established an ironworks in the 1640s. By 1700, Boston trailed only London as a ship-building city in the British Empire. "By the end of the Colonial era," [historian J. S.] Gordon writes, "the colonies were producing one-seventh of the world's supply of pig iron."
>
> As our Founding Fathers knew in their bones, this represented the merest beginning, situated as we were in what George Washington called "a most enviable condition."[61]

It is not surprising that a confabulation of wealth and salvation would produce a volatile mix so potent that it would sweep us along and into churning currents impossible to navigate given our limited vessels and systems. So buckle up and hold on!

Chrystia Freeland's article, "The Self-Destruction of the 1 Percent," compares the rise and fall of the Venetian fourteenth-century elite to the coming showdown with the 1 percent of wealth holders in the United States.[62]

Freeland, the editor of Thomson Reuters Digital and the author of *Plutocrats: The Rise of the New Global Super-Rich and the Fall of Everyone Else*, shares Thomas Jefferson's assessment of the economic structure alluded to in the Founder's era:

---

[61] Rich Lowry, "Pilgrims Planted the Seeds of America's Abundance," *Real Clear Politics*, November 26, 2009.

[62] Chrystia Freeland, "The Self-Destruction of the 1 Percent," *New York Times*, October 14, 2012.

In the early 19th century, the United States was one of the most egalitarian societies on the planet. "We have no paupers," Thomas Jefferson boasted in an 1814 letter. "The great mass of our population is of laborers; our rich, who can live without labor, either manual or professional, being few, and of moderate wealth. Most of the laboring class possess property, cultivate their own lands, have families, and from the demand for their labor are enabled to exact from the rich and the competent such prices as enable them to be fed abundantly, clothed above mere decency, to labor moderately and raise their families."

For Jefferson, this equality was at the heart of American exceptionalism: "Can any condition of society be more desirable than this?"

Freeland then proceeds to fast-forward to the present and portray our reversal of the democratic principles that brought us to where we are now. Before we leave her prescient analysis, I wish to call attention to another characteristic of governance relevant to the USA; that is inclusion versus exclusion:

The story of Venice's rise and fall is told by the scholars Daron Acemoglu and James A. Robinson, in their book "Why Nations Fail: The Origins of Power, Prosperity, and Poverty," as an illustration of their thesis that what separates successful states from failed ones is whether their governing institutions are inclusive or extractive. Extractive states are controlled by ruling elites whose objective is to extract as much wealth as they can from the rest of society. Inclusive states give everyone access to economic opportunity; often, greater inclusiveness creates more prosperity, which creates an incentive for ever greater inclusiveness.

That is vitally important for any empathic society and consistent with our commitment to the Golden Rule as an inclusive and enduring relationship catalyst. This could be applicable to both the secular and the sacred, with no conflict regarding the separation of church and state. We are focused on cooperation and understanding, all a part of our great heritage.

It is with this perception of our founding history that I wish to assign a more humanitarian import to what we call profit. Originating in Europe as early as the thirteenth century, it was disputed by the church, laboring under the stigma of usury, which was regarded at the time as forbidden by the Bible. The restriction applied by the Catholic Church was rolled back with the Protestant Reformation and their derivative creeds. In the mid-sixteenth century, Calvinism became the state religion of the Netherlands, which embraced its doctrine of predestination according to which certain devotees were presumed selected by God for salvation. A manifestation of this was demonstrated by success. This was regarded as corroboration that God had bestowed his approval and welcomed the devotee as a representative of his kingdom.

God Will Get It for You?

Acquisition and godliness appeared to converge from this traditional doctrine. The accumulation of wealth became a primary, visible, and revered feature, celebrated—conspicuously on display— though obviously, unfortunately, and, not unexpectedly, addictive. It may be a principal stimulant for that universal addiction to greed. The notion that one was selected by God should have sufficed, but the public pedestal was craved as well. Being influential among peers significantly elevated one's status in the community and further enhanced wealth-gaining potential. The off-the-precipice plunge into greed appears to be almost inevitable when a society embraces this sacred and secular blend of these symbols of celebrity, achievement, and divine selection. Hindsight has confirmed that one can appear holy and be hellishly selfish at the same time. Societal balance is difficult to maintain. This brief history helps clarify and adds perspective for the present.

Many of our laws appear, too often, to favor one group over another, with the more affluent consistently coming out on top. Mere chance cannot account for it. Lobbying is the means whereby the affluent continue their power. This intrusive ability to influence is one that borders conspicuously on bribery and that has been present but hardly accounted for. The similarity is more than symbolic or semantic. When practiced in excess it plunges us headlong into corruption. Corruption is to a sociopolitical system what complications are to a medical system, and all of this can be rectified by a healthy dose of transparency, ingested in the conscience several times a day, along with endless exposure. Concealment and deception are antithetical to a healthy democratic society. Whistle-blowing is hardly a good solution; it is like a risky medication with serious side effects. But it too is a symptom, and when it continues to pop up frequently, it could be telling us something important—and maybe we should be more attentive listeners.

Chapter Twenty-One

Golden Rule or Grand Exclusion

Consider the pursuit of inequality from the lofty, luxurious perches of the power brokers, who are busily designing systems of exclusion rather than inclusion. No nations or cultures are immune. No faith is challenged here. No deities, dogmas, or mythologies are offended. Historically, millions have died contesting their divisive differences. This is personal; it is about how we choose to treat one another. This is neither top down nor bottom up; it is universal. For a troubled and divided world, a very ancient antidote may be required: it is the perennial and globally respected social and behavioral equalizer commonly referred to as the Golden Rule.

The Golden Rule was incubated in synagogues, churches, mosques, and temples, and on the paths firmed by secluded holy men and philosophers, some dedicated, others detached, those who might have loved mankind but just couldn't stand the people. This rectifier and barometer of moral, ethical, and social truth remains cherished by most religions and spiritual movements, so it is nationally and culturally ecumenical. While many may regard this as utterly naïve or too nebulous or too ambitious a recommendation for our own complex society (referred to here as Wall Street, Main Street, and No Harm Street—three ineluctably converging intersections of capitalism, commerce, and cures), they represent the superhighways of our culture.

Often political discourse is studded with the clarion call, "We just need to go back . . ." We beckon our institutions, organizations, and systems to go back, way back—farther back perhaps than we have ever gone before. Nations, cultures, arts, and civilizations have disappeared, penetrated by the arrow of time, yet this maxim remains and is understood by all. Thus I make no apology for conceding an urgent need to draw on this very ancient universal statute of wisdom. Our world and our nation are now in dire need of simple sanity. This is a vital assertion: do unto others as you would have others do unto you. I am not calling for committees to convene and hammer out thousands of pages outlining numerous programs. This represents an age-old premise of social and personal cooperation and compatibility that would support a commendable unity for a healthy society—before anything else can be done.

Our decades-old penchant for facilitating institutional accessibility and harmony on a common standard, equitable for all, has had conversely a rather disturbing specter of idolizing greed. That is not working. Frequent wars—had enough of them yet? Religions, tragically, at least many, have come to embrace a prime directive mandating killing thy neighbors if they seem to disagree on most anything. And the lame protestation "but not ours" may be quickly dispelled by a brief but credible excursion into religious history.

As our three streets meet, taking from the poor to give to the rich, or vice versa, confronts us. None dare call it redistribution for fear of the "class warfare" stigma, though a more accurate euphemism for this slippery slope may be hard to pin down. I would drop those unnecessary labels and celebrate citizens working together for the benefit of all—inclusion not exclusion, celebrating equality rather than inequality. *Citizens United* comes to mind as a glowing concept. But that was snatched away by our Supreme Court, seemingly bent on pulling off an Orwellian caper. It depicts a country for sale to the highest bidders, where money is speech and corporations are people. That appears geared more toward fashioning a government of the billionaires, by the billionaires, and for the billionaires. They seemed to prefer the grand exclusion. "One person, one vote" was construed as tragically incompatible, for in a democracy all citizens are invited to speak, unsilenced, with their votes. It is time to come full circle by doing unto others equally. Want that city on a hill, one respected and emulated? A focus on the Golden Rule will bring us much closer than where we appear to be headed.

This is the model of social rectitude we boast, in this celebrated democracy, that we wish to have the world emulate. Now let's make it real. Many people worldwide would likely demur. Something is radically out of balance with that model if, while boasting openly of our commitment to equal opportunity, we are devaluing, gradually and systemically, the dignity of so many recently impoverished Americans.

We strive for our democratic ideal, equality of opportunity, a democratic axiom. This can conceptually translate into the Golden Rule of interpersonal behavior in a secular context or in a religious one for those who prefer it. Do unto others as you would have others do unto you, or briefly, do as you would be done by. We need to actively address this demonstrative disparity—the recent reallocation of wealth, and the inevitable resulting social inequality, which is now restricting social mobility and economic recovery. We best not boast too much about equality of opportunity, or our hypocrisy is apt to return to haunt us.

The Billionaire Cult

This is a bit of an oversimplification, but we have been worshiping wealth ever since we deluded ourselves into believing that God approved. But it just could be that we got it wrong, that God had nothing whatsoever to do with it, and that the Protestant Ethic was just one of those too-good-to-be-true-isms. Moving now from the sacred to the profane, consider this: An early example of the growing financial excess was the coming of the seventeenth-century tulip mania, in which we witnessed an early preview of the market boom and bust cycles One may refer to this cryptically as the "bloom" and bust cycle. Demand exceeded supply until the rotation went full circle and many delusional investors lost everything. We have been there and done that many times over—but the evidence of overindulgence in wealth continues to depict our excessive greed.

Lest this model appear a bit farfetched, we get a little help from—where else?—religion, as noted above. Remember, visible success via one's engagement in industrious work had come to be accepted as evidence that God had chosen the successful as one of the elect. The idea of being God's favorites or chosen by God was consistent with the doctrine of French theologian John Calvin, who became very prominent in our American heritage. Max Weber labeled it the Protestant Ethic in his 1905 book *The Protestant Ethic and the Spirit of Capitalism*. This influential work has, even to this day, given the accumulation of vast wealth a sacred dimension.[63]

If we think such backward dredging is like a reversed telescope, hoping that will bring visual clarity, bear with me for another peek. We now fast-forward to current characters—and no, this tale is not from

---

[63] Max Weber, *The Protestant Ethic and the Spirit of Capitalism* (1904) (New York: Routledge, Taylor and Francis Group, 2005)

a novel. Goldman Sachs, the world's premier financial institution, residing in the US, dipped its toes in the ethic discussed above to stave off some of the criticism for its unethical shenanigans (such as hoarding aluminum in Detroit, baiting customers as opposites, and profiting from both). The imagery returns to God and mammon. The CEO of Goldman Sachs, Lloyd C. Blankfein, described some of the more devious behaviors of this celebrated institution—because they were "successful"—as doing God's work. The fallout was not unexpected since Goldman had recently weathered a pretty unsavory history—more destruction than construction. In fact the *Wall Street Journal* brought this to us recently as a reminder. As I have suggested, this idea that it is acceptable to delude customers is apparently an ineluctably addictive philosophy because of what it portends culturally. That does not mean it is adaptive to our modern world; it may be we are just living in the distant past with witches, demons, and all, having changed only the costumes and semantics. Some of the early champions of this evolving movement did burn heretics at the stake, and they too are a part of our American religious tradition.

> Blankfein's wry comment that he's "doing god's work" seems almost to be a veiled jab at this sort of religio-public relations push, which to a serious banker of Blankfein's stature, must seem somewhat silly.
> Blankfein clearly knows who he works for. After all, God couldn't afford him.[64]

With God on the witness stand in this court convened for addressing God and mammon, deities and dollars, another mortal deserves to be heard: Sebastian Mallaby, whose forceful book is titled *More Money than God*. He presents the hedge fund movement as a

---

[64] Matt Phillips, "Goldman Sachs' Blankfein on Banking: 'Doing God's Work,'" *Wall Street Journal*, September 14, 2013.

vital and essential economic force in our current market. The book's title is flamboyant but revealing. The most successful managers make more than a billion dollars a year by feasting on market weaknesses, which they cleverly create and then passionately prey upon. He describes a dozen or so of these financial wizards, parading them before us with their lavish life styles. I will look briefly at just one: John Paulson. If Paulson was going to be a contrarian, he wanted to short something that could be totally wiped out. In the spring of 2005, he found his victim.[65]

> The target was mortgage securities, which combined every imaginable charm that a short seller could wish for. . . . The great American public had convinced itself that home prices could only go upward. . . . Banks turned these into mortgage bonds. . . . The most senior ones rated a solid AAA, the next AA, and so on to BBB and lower—there might be eighteen tranches in the pyramid. . . . But once nonpayments surpassed a 5 percent hurdle, the BBB securities would start suffering loses; and since the BBB tranch was only 1 percent thick, a nonpayment of 6 percent would take the whole lot of them to zero. . . . He paid $1.4 million for a year's worth of insurance, but if the securities were wiped out, he stood to pocket $100 million."

To make a long story short: John Paulson gambled big time and won many times over. And so goes the hedge fund feast. These managers made billions from unwary individuals, and finally taxpayers lost hundreds of billions of dollars. Mallaby's book is full of similar examples of people doing "God's work."

---

[65] Sebastian Mallaby, *More Money Than God: Hedge Funds and the Making of a New Elite* (New York: Penguin Press, 2010) pp. 327–28.

Transparency in Regulation

Hedge funds have certainly caught the attention of the regulators. They are keenly aware of and on guard against attempts to outfox the less fortunate by lobbying or other devious maneuvers. Their vocabulary, now familiar, has become standard fare on Wall Street: credit default swaps, collateralized debt obligations, and the ever-present derivatives. It is good to be reassured there is some serious effort to control these apostles of greed, especially since we continue to suffer from the effects of the 2008 financial collapse. Banks too big to fail are in effect manufacturers; the industry is hedge funds, and their product, billionaires. Many were so divested they will never return to normal.

A branch of government assisting in providing at least the appearance of regulation is the US Commodities Futures Trading Commission (CFTC). The most recent leader, Gary Gensler, has had extensive experience leading Wall Street firms (including Goldman Sachs for eighteen years). He also had previous experience in governmental financial administration, siding with those who were dedicated to deregulation—but that was prior to the 2008 disaster and his new responsibility to prevent it from happening again.

Recently, Joe Nocera, an op-ed columnist for the *New York Times* filled us in as to his identity and role as a game changer:[66]

When he came into office, the C.F.T.C.'s job was to regulate the futures market. It was a small agency, with fewer than 700 employees. Then came the Dodd-Frank reform law, which gave the commission enormous new responsibilities. It was charged with writing dozens of rules to regulate derivatives, and to oversee

---

[66] Joe Nocera, "The Little Agency That Could," *New York Times*, November 15, 2013.

a $400 trillion market. "I hadn't realized how much authority was delegated to regulators," he said. But he embraced the challenge. Derivative trades had always been conducted in the shadows; Gary Gensler brought them into the light.

"Today there is the modern version of a ticker tape, with the price and volume of every transaction," he says. "There is transparency in the market. That is what I'm most proud of." One of the scariest aspects of the financial crisis was that the government had no idea, for instance, that A.I.G. held a giant portfolio of credit default swaps that were poised to blow up the financial system.

Although the banking industry pushed back hard against some of the new rules, Gensler says that there was nothing radical about the new transparency. "Adam Smith wrote that the community at large benefits when you can make information and access free."

While this regulator might be helpful because his extensive experience in the business has given him insights into how to prevent the wealth manufacturers from stepping too far over the line, there are others who have crises of conscience and choose, because of their sensitivity, to do the unthinkable and pull out. One such person is Sam Polk, who told of his struggle recently and the crucial experiences that sent him packing. He had made a fortune by most anyone's standard but began to focus on the system he was using to acquire it and what that system was doing to most everyone else. Keep in mind our emphasis on how systems can corrupt good people. A brief excerpt from his account follows:[67]

But in the end, it was actually my absurdly wealthy bosses who helped me see the limitations of unlimited wealth. I was in a meeting with one of them, and a few other traders, and they were talking about the new hedge-fund regulations. Most everyone on Wall Street thought they were a bad idea. "But isn't it better for the system as a whole?" I asked. The room went quiet, and my boss shot me a withering look.

---

[67] Sam Polk, "For the Love of Money," *New York Times*, January 19, 2014.

I remember his saying, "I don't have the brain capacity to think about the system as a whole. All I'm concerned with is how this affects our company."

I felt as if I'd been punched in the gut. He was afraid of losing money, despite all that he had.

Mr. Polk reflected on the 2008 financial crash in this context, and how Wall Street had profited as they destroyed the less fortunate and then reaped lavish bonuses while those who were "too big to fail" walked away with billions in taxpayer bailouts. The immorality of it all got to him. Some people care about that.

Healthy, Wealthy, and Wise

If evidence of profit had symbolic influence pertaining to the life hereafter, it certainly carries a double whammy given the decisive influence on life in the here and now. Nowhere is this more significant than in its role in the health care so vital to all our lives. Money, medicine, and health take on a pertinent and ineluctable convergence.

The attempt to make health and medicine an exclusively economic issue will not do. That is short on social and community practicalities. My health and that of my neighbor are too interrelated, too inextricably interdependent, to ignore. It is a moral issue first and foremost, and our social structure will be adversely impacted by a restrictive philosophy that says, "You get good care only if you can afford it." Dangerous viruses and bacteria mutate and spread without our expressed consent. The harmony derived from compassionate inclusion and mutual caring is an umbrella of protection that benefits all of us. A healthy society is impeded by rationing health care; it must serve all of us, not just those who can afford it.

Viruses and bacteria are hardly class-conscious. The enormous resources we have spent, at times squandered, on terrorist hysteria, only to put in dismal performances in our encounters with hostile microorganisms, leaves us exposed to the devastating potential of epidemics. This is not too surprising, however, considering the lapses we exhibit in maintaining our infrastructure; by most accounts it is tragically depleted. Our leaders are busily preoccupied in their obsession with being perpetually reelected and then lobbying when they exit office in order to make enormous sums of money from the knowledge gained in serving their country. On the presidential level, we spend much of our time and energy three years in advance—while our country falls apart. Our sights are either absurdly long-term (our eyes on the next life) or obsessed with a short-term market millisecond. There is nothing left for the functional, practical earthly calendar of tomorrow, next week, or next year—or even the next ten years—by any calendar, from the Gregorian to the Hijri.

Chapter Twenty-Two

Profits over Patients

Your assumptions are your windows on the world. Scrub them off every once in a while, or the light won't come in.
— Alan Alda, actor and director (b. 1936)

There is an abundance of information available as we dissect the anatomy of profit's ascendancy in health care. This raises the fundamental question about the democratization of health services and the role money plays in pushing our society further down the path of inequality. This dynamic is seen most dramatically in the abundance or paucity of life-sustaining health services and their distribution within the population.

Profit is winning. Investors say it is a way of keeping score, but when winning is everything—meaning profit is paramount—one will do anything to win. It does help, as we look back, to determine how we got this way.

According to the ways of Wall Street, money "makes you do things you don't want to do." Or so goes the adage from the movie *Wall Street*.

Sampling various approaches to capitalism is in order. Capitalism means a variety of different things to different people. Over the years, we have come to realize that even the noblest attempts to institutionalize the sacred and the secular can and will be corrupted unless incessant vigilance is called upon to monitor both our intentions and actions. The absurdities are apparent as one of the most celebrated popes of the twentieth century calls capitalism to task, as reported by Maureen Dowd:

> After Communism collapsed, John Paul offered a stinging critique of capitalism, presciently warning big business to stop pursuing profits "at any price."
>
> "The excessive hoarding of riches by some denies them to the majority," he said, "and thus the very wealth that is accumulated generates poverty." [68]

To the good pope's observation, I would add this: It certainly does, and that is intentional. How else can the plutocrats stratify the social classes in order to fulfill their goal of having obedient and malleable multitudes to fight their wars, toil with marginal compensation in their businesses, and respond to most every whim the very rich choose to initiate and presume to deserve via their self-proclaimed status?

In keeping with the above papal conundrum, this is only the tip of the iceberg. Among the half dozen largest and most influential financial institutions, corruption is rampant, and it appears it is only recently coming close to being challenged by the attorney general's office. Capitalism and corruption may become synonymous.

In a post for the *Next New Deal*, the Roosevelt Institute's blog, Bruce Judson explains:[69]

> Unequal enforcement of the law will distort and destroy any capitalist society, and we may be witnessing just such a downward spiral in the financial sector representing Wall Street.

---

[68] Maureen Dowd, "Hold the Halo," *New York Times*, April 24, 2011.

[69] Bruce Judson, "For Capitalism to Survive, Crime Must Not Pay." *Next New Deal* (blog), Roosevelt Institute, April 12, 2012.

Capitalism is not an abstract idea. It is an economic system with a distinct set of underlying principles that must exist in order for the system to work. One of these principles is equal justice. In its absence, parties will stop entering into transactions that create overall wealth for our society. Justice must be blind so that both parties—whether weak or powerful—can assume that an agreement between them will be equally enforced by the courts.

There is a second, perhaps even more fundamental, reason that equal justice is essential for capitalism to work. When unequal justice prevails, the party that does not need to follow the law has a distinct competitive advantage.

The title of this blog post, "For Capitalism to Survive, Crime Must Not Pay," insinuates that our system of economic justice has put our society in jeopardy. This is not at all exaggerated. Consistently, we have seen "too big to fail" corporations benefit from the notion that they are too big to jail—so much for equal justice. The bailed-out banks brought back from the brink appear to have no fear of our legal system even though apparent crimes were committed. In order to function, capitalism requires a system governed by the rule of law. What the above states eloquently is that we have failed to provide the administration of law to assure the economic justice that capitalism requires.

In that abandonment of justice we have inadvertently jeopardized the coveted financial system we hail as a pillar of the foundation of America's greatness. As Chrystia Freeland explains in her *New York Times* article, "The Self-Destruction of the 1 Percent":[70]

That was the future predicted by Karl Marx, who wrote that capitalism contained the seeds of its own destruction. And it is the danger America faces today, as the 1 percent pulls away from everyone else and pursues an economic, political and social agenda

---

[70] Freeland, "Self-Destruction."

that will increase that gap even further—ultimately destroying the open system that made America rich and allowed its 1 percent to thrive in the first place.

Capitalism's Moral Compass

Capitalism unregulated is cannibalistic; it then destroys more than it creates. With each passing failure to prevent corruption and exercise the rule of law, accountability is deprived as we move ever closer to the precipice.

There is no invisible hand to make economic sense of this loss of a moral compass.

Profit, which is central in this system and vital in our history, becomes an irrepressible wrecking ball.

As we have noted above in tracing America as a youthful nation, profit, capitalism's primary endeavor, appears to be in our DNA. However, if corruption is legal, via selective enforcement, the balance of incentives for energizing our economic system will self-destruct. Our democracy, including the importance of medical equality, is our goal as a compassionate and caring nation. Children must not suffer if a family has no means of providing medical care when it comes to our life-sustaining health enterprise. As we assess the worthiness of engaging this issue, we are challenged to be clearheaded with our agenda.

Profit Plague

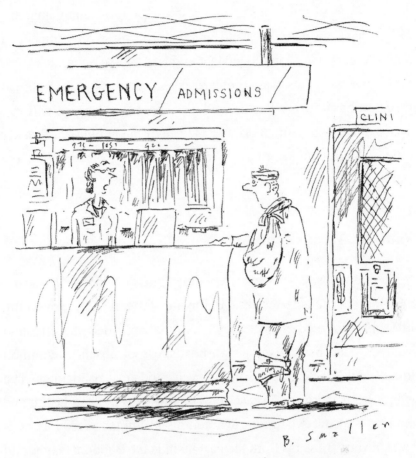

"There will be a bit of a wait while we figure out a market solution to your problem."

   CEOs have to maximize their companies' profits; it is their duty to shareholders, so our country is in fact for sale daily, to the highest flash bidder. Nationalism gives way to capitalism. The objective is now pure profit, uncontaminated by moral and ethical constraints. Gotta do what you gotta do! It's the ultimate demise of idealism, only this time it is not imaginative film fiction—it's the nightmare we fear.

We can't keep our finger in this dike. There would not be enough sandbags, even with sand from all our beaches, to hold back the rising tide. The oligarchs' billions cannot restrain the threatening anarchy. We will have no place to stand or hide. The disastrous impact of political corruption championed by our guardian, the Supreme Court, should give all of us pause, regardless of ideology. Any political office now has its price. Pay up, and it can be yours. This is a national disease, incurable without risking the life of the patient—a disaster in the making. One has to ask, did the Supreme Court really know what it was doing?

Common Misperceptions

The conquest of disease is, in the long run, protection from our most perilous enemies. Eclipsing fundamental governing philosophies (e.g., democracy, nationalism, secularism, and socialism—the basic -isms) may not take root absent a common outlook and the decline resulting from predatory pandemics. The ravages from scores of diseases can lay waste to life and health and could present overwhelming distractions to human reason as does abject poverty. Lessons from the past include the Bubonic Plague and flu pandemics. This overwhelming devastation and loss of life would prevent the implementation of these broadly organizing structures. It would be difficult to exceed basic tribalism and advance to envision nationalism, let alone entertain the individual equality found in a democracy highly dependent on sustaining the requisite foundational institutions.

Elevating our community to the vision of serious reflection means that orderly planning, resources, and commitments must be prioritized and redirected. Here we must become serious thinkers. There is a lot of money (profit) in war and a lot of money (profit) in medicine. Other people should not be regarded as our most formidable enemy. That portrayal is an insidious diversion, fueled largely by greed in support of the machinery of war. Eliminate the profit from war, and most wars will fade away. If we eliminate war against our fellow humans and instead target killer diseases, we establish exactly what should rise as targets for our attention and elimination. These diseases can then become the principal enemies on all fronts. Becoming internationally united in the pursuit of health and wellness is exciting to contemplate.

In some areas, we have relegated to charities the essential funding for vanquishing disease. This seems to be a tragic underestimation of need resulting in a misappropriation of resources, but it is consistent with the level of our value confusion. We should be glad to have the services the good charities provide for noble endeavors. But leaving medical care to charities reveals a tragic and misguided focus, failing to recognize our need as a nation. It may soon be conceivable that we suffer an international problem and thus recognize common enemies among the diseases that plague us all and join forces in pursuit of their control and elimination. Enlisting the United Nations in the pursuit of health appears to be a worthy undertaking whose time has come. The politics of this project could recruit the best minds in pursuit of international cooperation. I realize the old standby "nothing must ever be done for the first time" might be an obstacle, but this is worth thinking about.

Generous funds should be appropriated to eradicate the diseases that ravage mankind. These are the real killers and may even compete with Wall Street for the most talented soldiers of fortune. The profit issue enters here since we have spent (exhausted) our resources killing other people who differ from us. If we survive as a species, it will be in large part because we have come to understand our real enemies and strive to prevail over them. The polarization should not be in the ideological trivialities that we have chosen to focus upon. Race, religion, customs, culture, geography, and so on must not be automatic dictates for hostility. This is vital in our focus on the Golden Rule, an interpersonal governing philosophy for our democratic systems. The destruction of those with whom we disagree leads down that perilous path of self-destruction. (I expand on this in the epilogue and carry this premise to an interesting and challenging conclusion.)

Medicine's Mercenaries

Profits are sacred. If restoration surgeries and treatments were no longer profitable, the profit incentive would demand dramatically improved performance and a reduction in the number of repetitious procedures. Killing patients is one thing; losing money for private equity investors is almost unforgivable. That's killing the business. That this issue merits such consideration is in itself disturbing, as it borders on a system of cultivating medical mercenaries. Which is the more important of the two: profits or patients? Shouldn't this forever be a foregone conclusion?

As a result of this dichotomy, we see the potency of profits in our culture. This divergence of ethics contributes to medical concealment and the burial of mistakes, a horrible indictment challenging our basic humanity. Equating it ethically, bad incentives are a "moral hazard" (as Wall Street so euphemistically calls them), meaning that we are rewarding and thereby inviting disastrous performances that we do not wish to see repeated. This ranks very high on the harm index and should be regarded unequivocally as immoral and unacceptable.

Differences on these issues are seen in part as generational, which we shall see debated here.

In a recent *New York Times* piece, an Ivy League medical school student broached several issues percolating in the evolving medical system.[71] Incentives stood out when applied to medical practice and were found to be very offensive by some elder medical statesmen. Their efficacy was critically challenged as sweeping changes became more prevalent. These inserted motivators, good and bad, are now the hot topic of conversations on Wall Street, Main Street, and No Harm Street. Since the article was authored by Dhruv Khullar, a dual-degree candidate at the Yale School of Medicine and Harvard Kennedy School, where he is a fellow at the Center for Public Leadership whose studies and point of view represent his focus on both medicine and organizational management, it is pertinent in contemplating systemic change. Mr. Khullar concludes:

> As a student of health policy, I believe that incentives will be a powerful tool for changing physician, hospital and patient behavior—especially given the many perverse incentives that currently exist in our system. But as a student of medicine, I believe this focus on incentives must be coupled with an equally robust discussion of the historic and modern duties of a healer. We must promote a culture among students, residents and policymakers that recognizes that incentives—aligned, misaligned, askance or otherwise—are secondary to a physician's duty to fervently protect the health of patients.
>
> These two dialogues have largely operated in parallel, but it's time we integrate them and acknowledge their mutually reinforcing potential for delivering better care. Because alone, no arsenal of carrots and sticks will ever produce the kind of compassion and attention to detail every patient wants and deserves.[72]

---

71 Dhruv Khullar, "Medicine Is More Than Carrots and Sticks," New York Times, September 19, 2013.

72 Khullar, "Medicine Is More."

Generational differences moved quickly to the fore; some stalwarts in the medical community regarded their field as a "sacred calling," which from their perspective, provided sufficient inducement to fulfill the practical and routine duties in service of patients, absent incentives. The generational chasm was accented as mentors reminisced. As they recalled their decades of practice, the bygone days of yesteryear were deemed to have produced better medicine than what is currently emerging. Their experiences celebrated the superiority of a tradition they were reluctant to surrender. The system they embraced boasted a devotion to marathon routines, when thirty-plus-hour extended shifts were proof of intense dedication. There was little emphasis on current concerns regarding incapacitating fatigue, which evidence increasingly suggests brings with it the significant probability of grave medical errors. There was a noble emphasis on the redeeming value of sacrificing creature comforts, such as sleep and the routines of life surrendered to the calling. The mounting evidence of the urgent need for checklists and documented reminders to enhance patient safety was dismissed, and these measures were regarded as distracting intrusions. As I have pointed out, patients have died when inattention and disruptions resulted in essential tasks being ignored.

"To err is human" is an adage that obviously haunts those in the medical profession. Evidence is substantial concerning the value of practical procedures performed consecutively. There is proof that these procedures save lives. External monitoring, to check and double-check when lives are at stake, is now present in many professions that bear the noble burden of life-saving and life-sustaining work.

Relating this to my experience, medical errors were evident in sufficient number for me to question the potency of the supposed "sacred calling" and whether it is medically redemptive. One should not assume that the use of practical safety procedures has been embraced by even the majority of caregivers. Many appear to have no such commitment. Medicine is a noble and lucrative business. Given what we know, "trust and verify" should be increasingly applicable as a reasoned premise without debate. The medical community should insist on it.

What went irreparably wrong in my case, as evidenced via outcomes and repeatedly documented, should have been discussed openly. I believe concerted effort was exerted to limit my awareness of the full reality in order to prevent the assignment of accountability. This reaction is unfortunately systemic. The focus should be on changing that system rather than on extolling its virtues while denying its deficiencies.

The article to which I refer above is so recent that I feel its currency, coupled with the quality and source, is enlightening. Systems do not change easily, or quickly, nor without confrontation and controversy. Tradition, instead of digging in, may need to defend itself against these "perverse incentives," which must also go where the mounting evidence leads. There is too much of the undeserving "leave me alone to practice medicine as I please" attitude. Transparency will not comply.

I would remind the author of this article of the old adage: If it is eagles you want, you will need eagle eggs.

Fines: A Cost of Doing Business

A cost-benefit analysis could calculate the incentives needed to support system-wide models in order to facilitate planning and cover expenses for services provided. The balance of benefits and costs would assure a financially functioning system. Even penalties (fines) in many systems for patient neglect have been factored into the equation so the institutions can still turn a profit regardless of patient abuse. Our goal should be to have the medical profession plan from a patient-centered perspective, with the welfare of the patient prioritized over maximizing profits. We are striving for a patient-benefit analysis just as the investors would want for their own families—the Golden Rule premise.

Corruption in medicine has given it a reputation, unkindly, as a killing field, a system that must be closely monitored and in which criminal offences must be punished in the event of blatant violation of clearly stated regulations. That will be forthcoming only when those responsible are held accountable both financially and legally. Profit, that perennial motivator, when sacrificed, stirs and changes behavior like little else. Again, changes must factor in the cost of patients' medical restoration, including compensation for temporary or permanent behavioral interruptions, pain, and suffering, as well as other losses for which they should be fairly compensated. Now as the system rebels from within, hope is in the offing. Doctors and other medical professionals loathe the carnage of primarily profit-driven systems and are speaking out. It should be unacceptable to design a business model that profits after fines and flourishes in the process, while writing off penalties as a business expense and disregarding patient harm.

Profits and Purpose

Profits have a place in health care—as a servant, not a master. I have talked a lot about this because it is very important. Ailing patients must be treated and nurtured, and this treatment should not be based on how profitable a form of treatment is for private investors. Serving the health and well-being of the patient is crucial. The inordinate assignment of profits as a priority will result in the abdication of patient-centered priorities. Conflict of interest, if allowed to prevail, will dull the perception of the most astute diagnostician. Incentives must be central to the health of the patient and should serve that essential purpose. A medical system in which profit is paramount is a recipe for disaster. Serving the patient with a commitment to the restoration of his or her health is the goal that profit should help achieve. I continue to remind you of its importance because it dominates markets, businesses, and medicine without exception.

We are unveiling the dramatic influence of private equity investors on the functioning of a hospital chain and the resulting impact on doctor and patient relationships in the health care system that evolved.

> During the Great Recession, when many hospitals across the country were nearly brought to their knees by growing numbers of uninsured patients, one hospital system not only survived—it thrived. In fact, profits at the health care industry giant HCA, which controls 163 hospitals from New Hampshire to California, have soared, far outpacing those of most of its competitors. The big winners have been three private equity firms—including Bain Capital—that bought HCA in late 2006. HCA's robust profit growth has raised the value of the firms' holdings to nearly three and a half times their initial investment in the $33 billion deal.[73]

But as we shall see, the collisions of purpose manifest themselves as the policy, procedures, and delivery systems are calibrated for profits first, and the well-being of the patient is predictably diminished, according to many doctors. To meet the increased demands, safety

---

[73]   Julie Creswell and Reed Abelson, "A Giant Hospital Chain Is Blazing a Profit Trail," New York Times, August 15, 2012.

seems to have been sacrificed: Fatigue plagues the profession. Patient overload exists and concealment dominates as checklists are skirted. Leveraged buyouts by premier private equity firms are negotiated, and medical care is nearing the modern gold rush standard. Assuring profit dominance, even as neglect may include irreparable harm for which fines are levied, is the cost of business. Negotiate the penalties and settle for fines. As the money-and-morality dilemma unfolded, some doctors rebelled as they felt their practice was compromised.

> As HCA's profits and influence grew, strains arose with doctors and nurses over whether the chain's pursuit of profit may have, at times, come at the expense of patient care.
>
> Many doctors interviewed at various HCA facilities said they had felt increased pressure to focus on profits under the private equity ownership. "Their profits are going through the roof, but, unfortunately, it's occurring at the expense of patients," said Dr. Abraham Awad, a kidney specialist in St. Petersburg, Fla., whose complaints over the safety of the dialysis programs at two HCA-owned hospitals prompted state investigations.
>
> One facility was fined $8,000 in 2008 and $14,000 last year for delaying the start of dialysis in patients, not administering physician-prescribed drugs and not documenting whether ordered tests had been performed. .[74]

I wish to call your attention to a special report by *Time* magazine titled "Bitter Pill."[75] Many interested in medical costs have identified it as a must-read work and reference manual. The volatility reflected therein emerges with, among other things, exponential differences in costs for identical procedures and medicines from hospital to hospital.

---

[74] Creswell and Abelson, "Giant Hospital Chain."
[75] Steven Brill, "Bitter Pill: Why Medical Bills are Killing Us" (Special Report), *Time*, March 4, 2013.

Chapter Twenty-Three

Wall Street's Mythology

What "no harm" is to our health care system, the "Invisible Hand" is to Wall Street. Adam Smith could be called the prophet of Wall Street. He is credited, arguably, as coming up with a believable scenario in which the accumulated self-interest of society would be transformed into universal altruism when consistently indulged. This philosophical alchemy was brought about with the influence of a mythical Invisible Hand. Smith's followers, many of them titans of economic philosophy, curiously and repeatedly invoked this icon. By the press that it has generated in financial discourse, one could believe that it is a central theme in Adam Smith's work.

Justin Fox in his *Time* magazine column, "The Curious Capitalist," critiqued the odyssey of the Invisible Hand concept. According to Fox, Smith actually had little regard for the theory of the Invisible Hand. Wall Street, however, found it quite useful. Try to imagine the millions of dollars in bonuses this myth has generated! Here's how Fox puts it:

> You know Adam Smith for his "Invisible Hand," the mysterious force that steers the selfish economic decisions on individuals toward a result that leaves us all better off. . . . Lately, though, the invisible hand has been getting slapped. The selfish economic decisions of home buyers, mortgage brokers, investment bankers,

over the past decade clearly did not leave us all better off. Did Smith have it wrong?[76]

No, Smith did not have it wrong—but some of his self-proclaimed disciples have given us an incomplete and distorted picture of what he believed. The man himself used the phrase "invisible hand" only three times: once in the famous passage in *The Wealth of Nations* that everybody cites, once in another of his books, *The Theory of Moral Sentiments*, and once in a posthumously published history of astronomy (in which he was talking about "the invisible hand of Jupiter"—the god, not the planet).

Fox points out the following regarding *The Theory of Moral Sentiments*:

> Most of the book is an account of how we decide whether behavior is good or not. In Smith's telling, the most important factor is our sympathy for one another. "To restrain our selfish, and indulge our benevolent affections, constitutes the perfection of human nature."

Smith is describing a social relationship equivalent to the Golden Rule. He is very concerned with how we treat one another. A most revered economic philosopher finds a fundamental premise in generous reciprocity.

Justin Fox also demonstrates his own grasp of economic theory and practice in his award-winning best-seller *The Myth of the Rational Market: A History of Risk, Reward, and Delusion on Wall Street.*[77] Those who assume the "free market" has a deliberative, decisive mind and speaks coherently with an articulate, comprehensible

---

[76] Justin Fox, "What Would Adam Smith Say?" The Curious Capitalist, *Time*, March 25, 2010.

[77] Justin Fox, *Myth of the Rational Market: A History of Risk, Reward, and Delusion on Wall Street* (New York, HarperCollins, 2009), pp. 287–308.

message may wish to sample a bit of evidence that reduces it to the level of a casino. As an associate professor at Harvard and director of the Harvard Business Review Group, Fox has bona fides that give credence to his judgment and conclusions.

In a review of his book in the *New York Times*, op-ed columnist Paul Krugman says:[78]

> Wall Street bought the ideas of the efficient-market theorists, in many cases literally: professors were lavishly paid to design complex financial strategies. And these strategies played a crucial role in the catastrophe that has now overtaken the world economy.
>
> . . . Above all, he gets the way in which one's career, reputation, even sense of self-worth can end up being defined by a particular intellectual approach, so that supporters of the approach start to resemble fervent political activists—or members of a cult. . . .
>
> . . . Fox points out that academic belief in the perfection of financial markets survived the 1987 stock market crash and the bursting of the Internet bubble. . . .
>
> . . . And Wall Street's appetite for complex strategies that sound clever—and can be sold to credulous investors—survived Long Term Capital Management's debacle; why can't it survive this crisis, too?

Mythical Market Unmasked

We encourage those who embrace that approach to economics as a nonevolving science to be consistent. Why not have the same high regard for the practice of medicine, engineering, and cosmology as they were accepted nearly a hundred years ago? These have been surpassed as experience has modified theory. Where would the scientific contribution be without it? Could it be that the "rational market" we have worshiped lo these many years is quite irrational?

---

[78]   Paul Krugman, "School for Scoundrels," *New York Times, August* 6, 2009.

The more reasonable answer to the question "What is the market saying?" may be gibberish on occasion. One has difficulty worshiping profit as the prime directive when, after giving a fair hearing to its historic role in our culture, we find a good servant but a terrible master.

When I hear political persuasion exhorting passionately the need for fiscal austerity in a depressed economy, for example, I try to parse the logic of the argument. You'll discover that in the midst of what sounds like hardheaded realism (e.g., identifying an individual household budget as a parallel to government fiscal accounting) their ship of reason has run aground. "You wouldn't balance your checkbook that way," Someone might say. But the two are not parallel. In fact they are worlds apart. What works for one may be drastically dysfunctional for the other. The government economy gains momentum and benefits from spending collectively in our society; austerity drastically withholds what is actually needed and suppresses essential activity. One may reduce the speed of an airplane to the point that the wing taper, which enables the wind to compel upward thrust, can no longer resist the tug of gravity. Euphemisms are endless. Ask the local businessman at the cash register. My spending contributes to your income, and your spending contributes to my income. Real-world policies that will blight the lives of millions of working families are being guided on that plausible-sounding but erroneous premise—plausible because it is endlessly repeated and we can easily comprehend it. It is not miserliness but financial activity that creates economic health in a recovering and functioning, complex economy.

What deserves our skepticism, however, is the pursuit of universal self-interest, which has been transformed in our discourse into pure unadulterated altruism. Certain political persuasions seem to cherish ancient models echoing from the past, including elder political philosophers, some even feudalistic. If we are not careful, this could present a temptation for cherry-picking among classical texts to validate our own purposes. Time and social change, unless connected to more remote authorities, appear to be inauthentic to some. It has left the ardent adherents open to the often-quoted rejoinder that many of the great traditional champions were actually radicals in their own time and have been dead for a few hundred years! How relevant are they now in a global economy?

The Wall Street Sinkhole

The asphalt crumbled, and we all felt the fear of an horrific fall on that fateful day in 2008. The bubble sustaining our fragile economy was pricked, sending us into our worst economic disaster since the Great Depression. The titans gathered to see if enough fiscal cement could be pumped into that cavernous void to prevent the complete destruction of our and the world's economies. The panic was real, the threat, one of the worst imaginable. Wall Street collapsed!

In 2008 the *New York Times* editorial board laid out the problems:[79]

Finally, Americans need to be told a more fundamental truth: This crisis is the result of a willful and systematic failure by the government to regulate and monitor the activities of bankers, lenders, hedge funds, insurers and other market players. All were playing high-stakes poker with our financial system, but absent adequate transparency, oversight or supervision.

---

[79] Editorial, "Hard Truths about the Bailout," *New York Times*, September 20, 2008.

The regulatory failure, in turn, was grounded in the Bush administration's belief that the market, with its invisible hand, works best when it is left alone to magically self-regulate and self-correct. The country is now paying the price for that delusion.

The issue is one of access, and again transparency is postulated as a partial solution. It is easily demonstrated from the report above that Wall Street and No Harm Street are ineluctably joined and that their impact on our lives is inseparable. These streets are in desperate need of renovation.

It has become a fundamental failing at the core of our society. These flawed systems of capitalism and cures are driving debt, inequality, corruption, dissent, incompetency, and concealment, while at the same time generating multiple errors. Reform is essential because the corruption is crushing. We must adopt a new approach quickly, before vast infrastructure investments via private equity investors make corruption irreparable. Dramatic economic failure has extensive implications for our medical system.

Going Berzerk

Recall these recent reminders of how Wall Street imploded: On September 29, 2008, the market dropped 777 points, descending when the financial fiasco imploded our economy, plummeting into "too big to fail" territory, and revealing a financial catastrophe that proved devastating for our and the world's economies. This failure resulted largely from our leaders' complicit, intractable desertion of moral and arguably legal principles and financial realities calculated to enrich themselves and protect those complicit. The financial markets were left to the whims and shenanigans of those comparable to the robber barons of yesteryear. Legalized bribery took its toll. Backroom deals were arranged by the powerful and for the powerful, to ultimately benefit them and their corporations. The very next day a plan was contrived for an unparalleled bailout to help recover the damaged US and global markets. So as the banks were bailed out, our citizens were sold out.

We shall recuperate. It may take much longer, however, to restore the shattered trust. Serious harm has been done to our belief in the rule of law. Our ethical demise will be more lingering; broken trust is hard to heal. Hedge funds now rule the market and are known for instant money pursuits—and that will only increase the energy and time required to bring about a full recovery.

Casino Capitalism, Crony Capitalism, or "Free Market Capitalism"?

The fact that this criticism of unprincipled practice can be leveled by our most sophisticated and successful investors, legends in our time, speaks volumes regarding the damage inflicted on these pillars of our society. The social disruption and unheard of financial losses corroborate an unmistakable union of Main Street, Wall Street, and No Harm Street. On No Harm Street, we are horrified at the mysterious, imperceptible loss of human lives under the persistent systemic cloak of concealment.

Wall Street, however, had no place to hide; they could not bury their complications, try as they might, without burying the world's economy and sealing their own destruction. Focused transparency penetrated the financial market, revealing a system on life support from unbridled corruption. So stunning was this crippled economic structure that it was necessary for the president to address the nation in an ineffective attempt to quell the panic.

The chairman of the Federal Reserve was summoned to provide a prognosis and prescription. We had the likes of a delusional and critically ill patient, who lay in intensive care, attached to numerous supportive devices and monitored by overworked, traumatized, and at times inadequately prepared trauma professionals. The disaster was overwhelming. When causation was ferreted, reckless abandon was trumpeted from the stalwarts in our financial markets, who deplorably professed ignorance in order to renounce responsibility. They refused to be accountable. To have taken any responsibility would have saddled them with criminal intent. They would take ignorance and incompetency over criminality anytime—forget integrity and moral responsibility.

Plans for prevention must be addressed intelligently and sympathetically to sustain our nation's fiscal security and our citizens' sanity. Following the application of crisis support, efforts to recapture an emergency commitment to accountability were hastily approved. Cautionary measures were debated concerning a restoration design. Systemic sovereignty was challenged, with a call for monitoring behavior that appears to have been lackadaisical. At this point, there have been few if any changes in our nation's financial intuitions. This must never happen again, we vow, yet it appears we are setting up a replica of our recent implosion. Note the following examples, given our latest failures. Then stay on red alert, mindful of the truism that repeating the same behavior over and over while expecting a different result doesn't inspire our confidence.

Financial Bipolar Disorder

Thought it was over? On May 6, 2010, another market drop of seven hundred points precipitated by high-speed, millisecond trading and dubbed the "flash crash" again brought the country to a standstill. On August 5, 2011, a 512-point drop in the Dow was followed by a 630-point loss on August 8, accompanied by violent volatility never before witnessed in the "free market." If one attributed rationality to the market as some profess to do, it might have been characterized as having chronic bipolar disorder. That confusion is apropos, since the health of afflicted patients plummets as they neglect their prescribed medication, in this case (regulation) amid the reckless abandonment brought on by denial. Such behavior should not be—must not be—tolerated by our financial markets.

It is so like my experience in the hospital on a number of occasions—nobody appeared to be in charge while very important procedures were being planned and executed, putting the patient's life in jeopardy. Complex, integrated procedures requiring the utmost understanding and constant surveillance are necessary to assure optimal outcomes. The difference with the markets is that over a dozen participants are competing against each other in a win or lose scenario.

> A bad day in the stock market turned into one of the most terrifying moments in Wall Street history on Thursday with a brief 1,000-point plunge that recalled the panic of 2008.
>
> It lasted just 16 minutes but left Wall Street experts and ordinary investors alike struggling to come to grips with what had happened—and fearful of where the markets might go from here.
>
> At least part of the sell-off appeared to be linked to trader error, perhaps an incorrect order routed through one of the nation's

exchanges. Many of those trades may be reversed so investors do not lose money on questionable transactions.

But the speed and magnitude of the plunge—the largest intraday decline on record—seemed to feed fears that the financial troubles gripping Europe, which we largely provoked, were at last reaching across the Atlantic—and coming back home to roost. ...

Traders and Washington policy makers struggled to ride the bucking Wall Street bull and keep up as the Dow Jones industrial average fell 1,000 points shortly after 2:30 p.m. and then mostly rebounded in a matter of minutes...

But in the end, Thursday was not as black as it had seemed. After briefly sinking below 10,000, the Dow ended down 347.80, or 3.2 percent, at 10,520.32. The Standard & Poor's 500-stock index dropped 37.75 points, or 3.24 percent, to close at 1,128.15, and the Nasdaq was down 82.65 points, or 3.44 percent, at 2,319.64.

By the close, when calm was restored, the focus was on trying to understand what had happened.[80]

Bats in the Belfry

The opening and closing bells at the New York Stock Exchange herald both the beginning and closing moments. The ritualistic bell ringing is accompanied by applauding, enthusiastic participants focusing on the beginning or end of the day's financial activities. This ritual used to signify the precise opening and closing of market access. Since flash trading has now come to dominate the stock market, that appears to have been challenged. When the most experienced and successful Wall Street champions of the market unapologetically refer to our cherished financial system as "casino capitalism," "crony capitalism," or other such characterizations, they do so because of the close relation to No Harm Street and Main Street. This deserves our attention. It does indeed affect our way of life.

---

[80]   Graham Bowley, "U.S. Markets Plunge, Then Stage a Rebound," *New York Times*, May 6, 2010.

Confidence-shaking technology mishaps have been an almost daily occurrence at the nation's stock exchanges in the past few years.

A brief sample of the complications (recall that medical term indicating serious harm to the patient) was listed recently, a rundown of transactions that could not be smoothly or accurately processed. The list focused specifically on the BATS (Better Alternative Trading System), one representative sample of a dozen-plus systems committed to high-speed cyber warfare, with the ability to squeeze in profits from a millisecond advantage. The goal of the market in this system is to beat the competition with speed and volume. Profits accrue with the slightest difference—minuscule (pennies will do) for the preprogrammed trades—the superhighway to success in this chaotic market. Joe Ratterman, the CEO of BATS, was interviewed for an article in the *New York Times*, which disclosed these details:

> The latest example came Wednesday night when the nation's third-largest stock exchange operator, BATS Global Markets, alerted its customers that a programming mistake had caused about 435,000 trades to be executed at the wrong price over the last four years, costing traders $420,000.
>
> A day earlier, the trading software used by the National Stock Exchange stopped functioning properly for nearly an hour, forcing other exchanges to divert trades around it. The New York Stock Exchange, the nation's largest exchange, has had two similar, though shorter-lived, breakdowns since Christmas and two separate problems with its data reporting system. And traders were left in the dark on Jan. 3 after the reporting system for stocks listed on the Nasdaq exchange, the second-biggest exchange, broke down for nearly 15 minutes. . . . S.E.C. officials have acknowledged that they do not have adequate tools to properly police the high-speed, highly fragmented stock markets.[81]

---

[81] Eric Popper, "Errors Mount at High-Speed Exchanges in New Year," *New York Times*, January 10, 2013.

The suggestion that our financial architects may be a bit batty is perhaps merited.

The very recent turn of events on Wall Street render the critical issues we have addressed quite tame by comparison, yet they are vital to our understanding. Michael Lewis, well known for his monitoring of market integrity, has now stated openly that the market is rigged. Tremors from that recent declaration have been reverberating on Wall Street with aftershocks that have awakened or emboldened many critics. The market crash in 2008 and subsequent responses, some of which I have listed in this narrative, have left the average investor trembling on the sideline. A significant number of average individual investors either did not trust the market or felt they could not compete. That remains a significant loss to many hoping to use investment tools to help fund their retirements.

At my residence on Sunday, April 6, 2014, I viewed a *60 Minutes* segment entitled "Is the U.S. Stock Market Rigged?" and we can understand the repercussions. One of *New York Times'* serious financial critics, Joe Nocera, alluding to the program, writes:

> From where I'm sitting, it is a blessing that Lewis chose to write about high-frequency traders. Others may have come before, but nobody else could have created the firestorm that Lewis did by going on "60 Minutes" on Sunday and announcing that high-frequency traders had rigged the market. The F.B.I., the Justice Department and New York's attorney general, Eric Schneiderman, are now investigating high-frequency trading. The Securities and Exchange Commission, whose regulations unwittingly helped create the problem, is also said to be investigating. [82]

---

[82] Joe Nocera, "Michael Lewis's Crusade," *New York Times*, April 5, 2014. To investigate the *60 Minutes* narrative more fully, please refer to: CBS News, "Is the U.S. Stock Market Rigged?," http://www.cbsnews.com/news/is-the-us-stock-market-rigged/.

The arrival of "Flash Boys" has put a more important question on the table: whether high-frequency traders have been given an unfair advantage that needs to be dealt with. Lewis's answer is clearly yes, and "Flash Boys" is both clear enough and persuasive enough that Lewis's millions of readers are likely to agree with him."

Chapter Twenty-Four

Inseparable Pillars: Wall Street, Main Street, No Harm Street

Relationships involving this triad comprise the core societal configuration directing much of the traffic of our social systems. The cultural structure is evaluated financially, politically, ethically, and morally, encompassing the foundation of our independent community. Frequent contentions over budget constraints arise, along with demands for increasing quality and efficiency. This is particularly true of medical costs, which are now nearly 20 percent of our GDP, just about twice that of other Western democracies—double the money but not the performance, with little or no comparative enhancement. This raises serious questions, as it should. No Harm Street, for what we spend, should be a medical Autobahn by comparison. Experts tell us it is not, at least for the average Joe, for whom we seek a medical democracy. Data indicate we are lagging behind other countries. Challenges from Main Street and Wall Street urge reform. So what prevents our system from excelling to an extent that is commensurate with others on comparative costs? T. R. Reid has a lengthy career as a correspondent for the *Washington Post* and former chief of its London and Tokyo bureaus, and as a commentator for National Public Radio. Health care analysis is a priority for him. He has studied several countries, personally, as a patient, and offers his take, which is very enlightening. His assessment of good, better, and best will surprise most—it does not include our system.[83]

No-Harm Charm

Let's take a peek into the past by analyzing the celebrated "no harm" aphorism historically embraced and revered by the medical profession here and abroad. While the origin of the expression is uncertain, it appears to represent the philosophy derived from the Hippocratic Oath. Considering all aspects of progressive medicine, we should challenge the veracity of the oath as a constructive decree. It seems to represent an unproductive goal, as it is universally enshrined in medical tradition. It stands as a classic example of medical epigraphy. Exploring revered symbols can cause one to run the risk of appearing disrespectful, but my intention is to join a call to reform initiated by the awakened modern medical community, for the improvement of our system for patient care. Enhancing the inclusive quality of this service for all citizens continues to be our primary objective, one that is consistent with our growing democracy.

Once we move beyond the aura derived from repetitive use of the phrase, analysis becomes possible. Some evolving traditions can be very helpful. An acute awareness of where we have been can help us chart a course for the future. Our purpose is goal oriented and remains pragmatic; examination of historic struggles is instructive. Harry Truman's line is relevant: "The only new thing in the world is the history you don't know."

---

[83] T. R. Reid, *The Healing of America: A Global Quest for Better, Cheaper, and Fairer Health Care* (New York: Penguin Press, 2009), pp. 163–83.

No Harm Street: Bumpy and Expensive

On a more everyday level, I recover my auto (i.e., myself) from the "no harm" medical services department after bouncing about on the bumpy road of No Harm Street. The defect has not been corrected; the same threatening symptoms remain. I register a reasonable concern and am confronted with the equivalent of the "no harm" aphorism. I am assured it is really no worse than when I came in—no harm but no help. I am assessed full fees (which is indeed harmful) and sent on my way (further delay that represents further harm). They will have another go at it if I can get on their busy calendar for a distant appointment, but full fees will of course be necessary the next time around. Also, I may be required to post a copay (more harm) as I sign in—that is, before they will begin. All subsequent attempts will involve the same runaround whether improvement is achieved or not.

A layman delved into the analysis of the no-harm philosophy and rendered this pertinent observation: it was time specific. Essayist Chuck Klosterman, in his *New York Times* column "The Ethicist," argues that the use of the Hippocratic Oath is outdated, but he appears guarded in his modest support.

> But I feel that the first thing we need to recognize is that the Hippocratic oath represents the ideals of a person who died in the historical vicinity of 370 B.C. Now, this doesn't make it valueless or inherently flawed. It's a good oath. But we're dealing with a modern problem, so I would separate the conditions of that concept from this discussion.[84]

---

[84] Chuck Klosterman, "Should I Protect a Patient at the Expense of an Innocent Stranger?" The Ethicist, *New York Times*, May 10, 2013.

Klosterman addresses this veneration for a principle that has very little to do with present conditions, pointing out that it is really a bit out of touch with our modern twenty-first-century culture.

Contrast Wellness as Constructive and Directive

Fast-forward to practical applications, and the luster fades as absurdities rise. Many in and out of the profession are maintaining that "no harm" may be in fact harmful when applied.

From a practical perspective, consider how we might fare with our platitude if we used it to address international relations. Would historic international powers relating to one another just by avoiding actionable hostilities be regarded as exceptionally worthy? As a matter of fact, that dynamic would not even rise to the dignity of peace, let alone that of cooperation and mutual striving for progressive international accomplishments. Pursuit of outstanding endeavors may yet be achievable. Consider the benefits of planning together to build a more humane society with mutually approved standards applicable for all that consequently engender a more harmonious relationship. But No Harm Street projects an impotent, anemic nuance. Wellness is essentially positive, therapeutic, and directive, a basic evaluative criterion that is scientifically measurable. For nations, enhancing programs for the purpose of lifting citizens' prospects would be desirable and achievable.

My Too Recent Brush with No Harm

A longstanding love of tennis provided me with good exercise and enjoyable recreation. Most of my play was in the Southeastern part of the US, while my ancestry boasts of European descent, my ancestors hailing from cooler climes with less penetrating sunlight. My fair complexion, even with the best SPF protection, left me with lesions that from time to time were biopsied, with a verdict of squamous carcinoma. This of course involved minor surgery to prevent a major threat, always an essential procedure accompanied by a minor inconvenience with an interruption of routine activities. Several procedures conducted to extract lesions have yielded excellent results for which my family and I are very grateful. The dermatologist was remarkably skilled at suturing virtually without a trace. The most recent instance, however, which I am recounting for you, carried a surprise that left me, well, harmed.

In the previous encounters, the practice was to remove the offending tissue, and before termination of the procedure, conduct a lab test on site to immediately assure us of a complete eradication. This time around I had opted for and expected the same process, and was assured of such when I scheduled the procedure. My appointment day arrived and we entered at 7:35 a.m. I prefer to get unpleasant experiences over with ASAP, so I had intentionally scheduled the procedure for early in the morning. While I occupied the chair and was being prepped, the surgical assistant informed me that the process would require just one attempt but the results would not be available for a few days. I was a bit taken aback, but at that point, having undergone several successful surgeries there, I did not interrupt the process or ask further questions. It took less than an hour, and we were on our way.

I am an anemic senior citizen with a history of MRSA (a contribution from my earlier surgical experiences elsewhere). Even the biopsy for this procedure turned the MRSA red—amaranthine—and it spread aggressively. We treated it with Mupirocin ointment, which we keep on hand because of my vulnerability. After three days, the infection began to recede. I had been issued an antibiotic, Cephalexin, the day of the surgery. The dosage was 500 milligrams, three tablets per day, to be taken for a week to reduce the MRSA potential.

The recovery was uneventful with the exception of interrupting my workout routine, very important for me, and limiting other daily chores for fear of rupturing the sutures placed in my left forearm. My unfortunate da Vinci encounter in 2007, followed by abdominal surgeries for removal of adhesion-produced blockages, had resulted in the decimation of most of my abdominal muscles. That limitation necessitates the use of both my arms to navigate comfortably; eliminating use of one arm for the required three to four weeks was a serious disadvantage for me (though perhaps less so for others with no handicap). Since my abdominal muscles have been damaged by the essential follow-up surgeries, getting in and out of the car, rising from a chair, lying down and getting up, putting on socks and so on, all required the use of my arms for assistance. The risk of serious injury from falling is higher with these surgical limitations.

Elderly Independence

My wife and I also own and manage a small apartment business (a few dozen units). We hustle to keep the vacancy rate low. An unwritten perk for tenants completing a year with us is a $1,000 interest-free loan, available to them if the need arises. This benefit has helped several buy food and medicine on a number of occasions during difficult times. Maintaining this business helps prevent our being a financial burden, though it does require substantial supervisory and bookkeeping work on the part of both my wife and me.

My wife was diagnosed with Parkinson's disease over a dozen years ago. She has been extremely lucky inasmuch as it has progressed very slowly. She receives excellent treatment from her neurologist, who prescribes an effective cocktail of medications. She is also very dedicated to regular exercise routines, including the habitual practice of tai chi, a Chinese therapeutic exercise program recommended for Parkinson's patients.

Both my wife and I have found healthful support and improved freedom of movement through massage therapy. We are fortunate to have a highly skilled therapist recommend enthusiastically by a nationally renowned orthopedic surgeon.

We continue to reside in our spacious four-bedroom house, where we reared our three children. It has a beautifully landscaped yard (over an acre) where my wife delights in cultivating stunning flowers and assorted shrubs. We enjoy our well-equipped gymnastic sunroom. It has a multistation Vectra exercise assembly, a rack of dumbbells, a Lifecycle stationary exercise bike, a treadmill, an inversion table, and other assorted exercising paraphernalia. Our swimming pool, which measures eighteen feet by thirty-six feet and rests in view of the sunroom, was built for the children, and we still choose to retain it for its beauty and as a reminder of what it has meant in our lives.

My wife maintains the chemical balance in the pool, and I do most of the skimming. It is lovely and blends nicely with the well-landscaped terrain. Just skimming our pool to remove the rapidly falling leaves requires both arms, so repeated surgeries, if unnecessary, represent a real inconvenience. A friend visiting in our sunroom reminded me that our "sparkling pool" needed attention. I held up my arm, recovering from duplicated surgeries, and said: "It will recover, too; but in the meantime we may have to settle for fifty shades of green." I hope this detail helps you understand, in part, my reaction to the surprising surgical procedure described above.

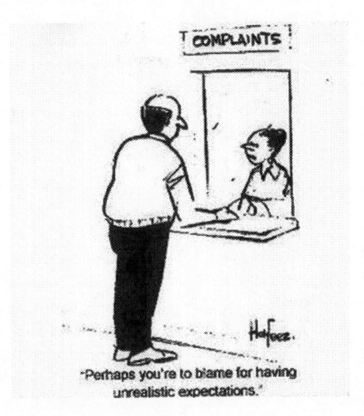

"Perhaps you're to blame for having unrealistic expectations."

A Failed Surgery

Within a few days of the procedure, I received a call from the dermatologist's office. They were sorry to inform me that I would have to repeat the surgery since they had not removed all the offending tissue. The young lady was very polite—but I was furious, and I let her know that. I felt guilty, as I have on one other occasion when the messenger on that end of an encounter shared unpleasant and controversial news. I asked to speak with the doctor and was told they would give him my message. I received a return call indicating the doctor would be in surgery all day. The call was returned by another staff member who said that in two weeks they would remove the existing sutures and then we could schedule the next surgery. I had a little concern here (related to my age and experience) regarding having back-to-back surgeries too soon, given the trauma to the body, the need for another round of antibiotics, and so on. This is far more risky for an elderly patient who may have additional issues than it is for a much younger and healthier person.

Patients and Procedures

The goal of patient-centered medicine takes into account the needs of an individual patient. That challenges the alleged superior stature of procedure-centered medicine, absent exceptions for individual difference, which we are addressing here. Procedure-driven applications having little flexibility may tend to be more rigid than medically practical for the patient's needs. In my case the stated rationale for implementing the procedure was their growing confidence in its first-time success rate. Their data, shared with me, was based on informal conversations that I had (not scientific) and revealed that only 2 percent of patients had to receive duplicate treatments. That small and, to them, insignificant number made their approach preferable for all patients. As this was being explained to me, I reminded the messenger that perhaps age, medical history, and other pertinent details might need to be considered as qualifiers rather than assuming a one-size-fits-all approach. It didn't matter if one were eighteen and in robust health or eighty (my age) with compromising conditions, the procedure was the same; it was procedure-centered rather than patient-centered. My use of the term procedure-centered has no reference to the exceptionally technical procedures that involve teams of highly skilled surgeons performing complex operations where vital organs are the target of therapy. But again, I was speaking with the messengers, not the deciders. An important justification, which I verified with the insurance provider, was that it had become insurance related; their approach was in compliance with their negotiated insurance coverage—and thus became what I will term "system-centered." I wonder if anyone professionally affiliated would consider an exception to this hard-and-fast rule if they were treating a member of their own family. Keep in mind we are working for a compassionate medical democracy.

My call to schedule the repeat surgery involved an interesting twist. As we worked on a date, it appeared we had to settle for a month's wait from the time of my call. I asked to be placed on a waiting list in case of a cancellation. A few days passed, and I realized that, in my file of carefully maintained medical notes, I did not have my up-to-date medical records from that office. I had them from all other medical providers. I called and requested a copy of my record. The office faxed a form for me to return. In less than ten minutes, a staff member called and invited me to take a cancelled appointment slot for the very next day at 12:40 p.m., which I gladly accepted.

We were treated very courteously, as always. I had not had an opportunity to speak with the surgeon since the controversial "need to repeat" phone call. And I have made it a practice, based on experience, to never engage a surgeon bearing a scalpel, on any controversial issue; it's not the time or the place. I'm serious—no attempt at humor here.

The surgery went as planned; the offending tissue was removed, and I was treated with a temporary bandage and invited to a waiting room with several other patients. After nearly an hour we were informed the test was negative. We were then called to the surgical room and prepared for the sutures. The surgical assistant started to remove the bandage with her bare hands, and I requested that she please put on gloves first. Beyond that little caveat, all went well. Our medical practice is not patient-centered. My dermatologist, is highly skilled and does excellent work. My dissatisfaction in most of these medical concerns continues to be with systemic issues.

If one were to examine this risk of double surgeries for a percentage of unlucky patients more thoroughly, these factors, among others, would be worth considering: Who did the research? Who funded it? What is the profit differential on the newer procedure? What are the negative side effects for those who get caught in that 2 percent net? What was the sample size of their study? My expertise in research design is very limited, but it seems this may deserve closer scrutiny.

In my recent reading, I came across a medical report that caught my attention, inasmuch as it referred to a related medical issue. Another patient of a dermatologist located halfway across the country had endured an incident that dwarfed my complaint. A small skin lesion on her cheek escalated into a triple-specialist encounter, several procedures, and enormous costs. This is not directly connected to my experience, but it is worth noting, as it may represent a trend.

In an article called "Paying Till it Hurts," writer Elisabeth Rosenthal describes the case of this woman, who had to endure surgery that resulted in a huge bill:[85]

---

[85] Elisabeth Rosenthal, "Paying Till it Hurts—The High Earners: Dermatology Patients' Costs Skyrocket; Specialists' Incomes Soar," *New York Times*, January 18, 2014.

"I felt like I was a hostage," said Ms. Little, a professor of history at the University of Central Arkansas, who had been told beforehand that she would need just a couple of stitches. "I didn't have any clue how much they were going to bill. I had no idea it would be so much."

Ms. Little's seemingly minor medical problem—she had the least dangerous form of skin cancer—racked up big bills because it involved three doctors from specialties that are among the highest compensated in medicine, and it was done on the grounds of a hospital. Many specialists have become particularly adept at the business of medicine by becoming more entrepreneurial, protecting their turf through aggressive lobbying by their medical societies, and most of all, increasing revenues by offering new procedures— or doing more lucrative ones.

For her follow-up, she refused to return to Baptist Health and went instead to the University of Arkansas Medical Center, where a dermatologist told her she likely had not needed such an extensive procedure. But that was hard to judge, since the records forwarded from Baptist did not include the photo that was taken of the initial lesion.

The photo should have been required. Transparency will advance the medical system for the good of all.

My advice for older or compromised patients: you are aware of those special needs, others may overlook them. Keep in mind, this is a business. All other things being equal, take your medical concerns to a provider who will make adjustments for your special needs. I try to continually remind myself that our dedicated medical professionals are not villains. They are very good people; it's the system that is broken.

This parallel is not perfect, yet the absurdity is evident and shocking once you see the process by comparison. I have tried not to exaggerate my own treatment when put beside standard medical practice. It is at times a minimalist service credo, and medically, it deserves to be reevaluated. One should not be rewarded for "no harm," which is really harmful (to my bank account as well as my health). I am poorer as a result, have been harmed, and have lost precious opportunities. Positive results need to be incentivized, and "no harm" regarded as an antiquated goal. A failed attempt at a cure is in fact harmful in most cases. In addition to suffering through further invasive injury, the patient endures the loss of time, opportunity, endurance, health, and money. And the patient's potential for healing is usually reduced with each repeated "no harm" surgery.

Dr. Makary has confronted numerous weaknesses in the medical system. In the *Wall Street Journal*, he challenged readers with the headline "How to Stop Hospitals From Killing Us." This serious charge by a renowned medical insider is sobering.

> Many Americans feel that medicine has become an increasingly secretive, even arrogant, industry. With more transparency—and the accountability that it brings—we can address the cost crisis, deliver safer care and improve how we are seen by the communities we serve. To do no harm going forward, we must be able to learn from the harm we have already done.[86]

As Dr. Makary states, the concept of "no harm" as a change agent has turned out to be an appallingly unacceptable incentive. Wall Street introduced the concept of "moral hazard" to describe and deter irresponsible compensation for unsavory endeavors. Do not continue to pay for behaviors you do not wish to have repeated. They were in effect stating that bad incentives evoke moral deviousness. It is time for medicine to move beyond its mythical past and reinvent itself too, time to harvest the cumulative benefits of revolutionary,

---

[86]   Marty Makary, "How to Stop Hospitals From Killing Us," *Wall Street Journal*, September 22, 2012.

evolving medical science. Just in recent years astounding advances in DNA, stem cells, the genome, and regenerative medicine, to cite a few milestones, indicate the astonishing possibilities on the horizon. There is little time and no place for the old "no harm" myth.

Turning onto No Harm Street, shrouded beneath antiquated ideologies, blind to the realities of the secluded medical practices, lies another vital system run amuck. We can and do, quite literally, bury our medical mistakes by the thousands. These are not anonymous strangers: they are our children, our parents, ourselves!

Must Pretend—It's Expected

These aspiring professionals are in the most competitive field imaginable and feel pressured to feign required skills they have not yet acquired. Immediate execution of very difficult procedures, absent the requisite experience, talent, and ability, seems to be a part of an unwritten code referred to frequently by medical professionals. This expectation, conveyed subtly, motivates aspiring participants to risk faking skills they have yet to attain, thus risking injury to unsuspecting patients on whom they must then perform these elusive procedures. Let's construct a hypothetical example to explore this dilemma. See it, do it, pass it on to another quickly—this is in-service training via the medical model alluded to. Translating that scenario into athletic terms, one might imagine having to achieve some acrobatic skill with minimal exposure, always needing to get it right immediately to perpetuate the mythology. If seeing it is acquiring it, all the extraordinarily talented intern must do is follow the expert after a brief exposure. Acapulco cliff diving—a breeze on the first try. Just follow the expert diver off the precipice after you watch her demonstrate. Then having just acquired the skill, return and demonstrate the remarkable talent to another trainee and watch him follow you off the same cliff. The recently inducted trainee will then pass it on to another, a scenario repeated ad infinitum. Scamper across Niagara Falls on a high wire—you name it, they can do it instantly—and what's more, successfully instruct most any newcomer who may be in training and expected to perpetuate the myth. Isn't this a model for disaster? I have deliberately chosen examples where the risk is on the neophyte helping to expose how unconscionable this practice is; owning the danger may help to inject rationality into this atrocious model. Such unrealistic expectations, whatever purpose is intended, would quickly vanish in the light of transparency. The sooner, the better, for the sake of the patient and the integrity of the medical model.

The profession, living up to the myth, expects too much, too soon, and patients are injured and killed, victims of this rite of passage—hardly a character-building experience. Would the students or faculty expose members of their families to this high-wire act of high-risk medical practice? We really care about our medical professionals in training. We need their brilliant minds, exceptional skills, and moral integrity.

Beware of the myths—they are little more than lies dressed up in tuxedos. We have innumerable myths parading in our modern world, dragging the cumbersome chains of a barbaric past that must be quickly outgrown.

We are inundated with images of the astounding medical miracle worker, whose silhouette dominates, daily, on prime-time TV shows and commercials. We are presented with an omniscient, tireless performer, routinely pulling twenty-four- to thirty-six-hour shifts, then arising fresh and ready to practice faultless medicine with only a modicum of rest. In reality, from our experience and what we have learned from the medical professionals' confessions and disclosures, an unwitting potential killer is on the loose. This indefatigable modern super saint is consecrated by expectations and related promotional endeavors to construct an image of one who deserves unquestioned commitment and loyalty—but that image is rapidly wearing thin.

Thanks in part to deliberate rationing by the profession, which is likely economically driven, we have an alarming shortage of qualified doctors even in the face of the demands and needs of our growing complex system and aging population. The crisis will escalate. But we can expect substantial resistance to any maneuver that could possibly interfere with the steady rise of the wealth quotient surrounding the medical profession. That resistance is to be expected from any challenged and lucrative business, even more so from one that has inherited and perpetuated a comparable degree of self-adulation. Members of the medical community comprise a substantial political power base in our society, a position from which they brandish incalculable influence.

With the veil of invincibility pierced, fallible human providers come to visualize themselves under a persistent threat of malpractice costs with career-threatening implications. As patients grow more restive and demand compensation for the profusion of serious medical errors, and as the doctors bear the cost in pain, suffering, and resources, change may become possible. A handful of prominent academic medical centers, like Johns Hopkins and Stanford, are trying a disarming and refreshing approach to systemic change. In addition, as we have seen in this book, numerous medical professionals are breaking with the concealment philosophy and opening up in their books and journal articles, urging transparency as a means of reducing that destructive mythical aura.

This change will boost medical science. With so much to learn—and now so little to hide—they can explore and innovate at a pace that accelerates exponentially. Patients' role as contributors will help mitigate the anger that fuels many of the lawsuits. Malpractice lawyers say that what often transforms a reasonable patient into an indignant plaintiff is less the error than its concealment, which fuels the victim's justified concern of harm done and that it will happen again.

Reformers hope that, by promptly disclosing, rather than hiding, medical errors and offering sincere apologies and fair compensation, they can raise the level of trust regarding the care of patients, make it easier to learn from mistakes, and diminish the anger that often leads to destructive litigation.

Chapter Twenty-Five

Follow the Money

If money be not thy servant, it will be thy master. The covetous man cannot so properly be said to possess wealth, as that may be said to possess him.

—Francis Bacon, essayist,

philosopher, and statesman (1561–1626)

Given our tolerance for mediocrity, or even deficient outcomes from the past, to expect an immediate leap to excellence is to refuse to acknowledge what we know of human nature. The system needs changing, and friendly forces are now emerging from within to accommodate a serious attempt. Our resistance to change is perennial, yet at the same time, we expect more favorable outcomes. Systemic change is going to require accountability and verification on several levels, top to bottom and bottom to top. This calls for a penetrating transparency. Money is writ large on the entire package, as our marriage of money and medicine reveals. There are no prenuptial agreements here. The conflict between Wall Street and Main Street, to a degree, underscores the recent hijacking of our traditional "free market," which average folks used to rely on for retirement and financial security. Wall Street has effectively killed it and thereby convoluted the potential democracy of medicine. Wall Street's elitism impacts all three streets, with No Harm Street being most closely affiliated organizationally with Wall Street.

I must confess part of the title of one particular article, "With Money at Risk . . ." riveted my attention and compelled me to read it. The ones at risk were obviously the patients whose safety was compromised. As I have learned, as this book explores, and as my experience and research confirm, health care cannot be understood in America without focusing on its intriguing relationship with Wall Street. That is why I have addressed this connection so thoroughly.

> At North Shore University Hospital on Long Island, motion sensors, like those used for burglar alarms, go off every time someone enters an intensive care room. The sensor triggers a video camera, which transmits its images halfway around the world to India, where workers are checking to see if doctors and nurses are performing a critical procedure: washing their hands.

It becomes more appalling as it goes. Alarms and bells signal around the world, at the speed of light. We are assessing the life-and-death issue of simple hand hygiene and the difficulty confronted by cajoling and imploring the treating professionals regarding the necessity of their washing their hands to avoid contaminating patients with deadly bacteria and viruses. As the author points out, they fail to do this about 70 percent of the time; and doctors (No Harm Street's highest-ranking officers) are the worst offenders. The hospitals have adopted near-CIA tactics. Coaches and cameras failed to enforce the simple procedure. If my summary sounds severe, listen to their enforcers:

> "This is not a quick fix; this is a war," said Dr. Bruce Farber, chief of infectious disease at North Shore. . . . But the incentive to do something is strong: under new federal rules, hospitals will lose Medicare money when patients get preventable infections.

Of course we are back to the money again.

It was noted that patients' families would inquire about whether hand washing had been done, so the author said, and it was because they understood the risks. My observation from experience is that it was because they cared. The medical professionals appeared not to. Were they callous or ignorant? That is an embarrassing question. Perhaps a more ameliorative conclusion can be drawn; but this invites infection, and that is a killer. The article concludes with a more disturbing and somber note:

> Dr. Larson, the hand-washing expert, supports the electronic systems being developed, but says none are perfect yet. "People learn to game the system," she said. "There was one system where the monitoring was waist high, and they learned to crawl under that. Or there are people who will swipe their badges and turn on the water, but not wash their hands. It's just amazing."[87]

Yes, it is amazing but, judging by my experience, not at all exaggerated. This simple yet essential hygienic ritual seemed to be violated repeatedly in every medical institution in which I was a patient, and I have alluded to it on several occasions.

Maybe the mysterious "invisible hand" needs to be washed on Wall Street as with medical professional's hands on No Harm Street, using a detergent to banish greed and germs and instill trust. Until then, we must verify!

---

[87] Anemona Hartocollis, "With Money at Risk, Hospitals Push Staff to Wash Hands," *New York Times*, May 28, 2013, http://www.nytimes.com/2013/05/29/ nyregion/hospitals-struggle-to-get-workers-to-wash-their-hands. html?nl=todaysheadlines&emc=edit_th_20130529.

Hospitalist to the Rescue

My emergency admission to the hospital ER, prompted by bowel blockage, was very frightening, even when repeated multiple times. Routine checks, followed by the dreaded insertion of the nasogastric (NG tube), are experiences one never forgets. Nasogastric aspiration is frequently used to remove internal blockages. But there is no way to minimize the discomfort of having that tube thrust in your nostril, down your throat, and into your stomach, to relieve the pent up-pressure by extracting the contents of your digestive system. On April 5, 2011, the medical staff attending to me at the ER appeared tentative and inexperienced at effective insertion of the tube. Five attempts by three different staff members were made over a couple of hours—an eternity—to no avail.

I'm an NG Guinea Pig?

A neatly clad gentleman in formal medical attire, his white coat sharply creased, strode into the room with a confident manner and relieved a flustered assistant who had made two previous attempts at my NG procedure. In less than thirty seconds he had the tube in place and secured by a strip of tape on my nose. He, self-assured and assertive, identified himself as the physician in charge of my care. Now, after having read a dozen books and several journal articles, I am not surprised at the assistant's floundering behavior. After only brief instructions for medical practitioners (brief because, as noted earlier, there is the economy of time, and equally important, there is the need to maintain the myth of proficiency and competency reflected in acquiring skills with little exposure—they learn so quickly by doing), they are expected to master tasks rapidly. I speak from painful experience. It's a myth that partly trained personnel can master procedures so easily. They often learn at the patient's harm, following serial failures.

The hospitalist has emerged as a new player on the medical stage. According to the Society of Hospital Medicine (http://www. hospitalmedicine.org/), a hospitalist is "a physician who specializes in the practice of hospital medicine. Following medical school, hospitalists typically undergo residency training in general internal medicine, general pediatrics, or family practice, but may also receive training in other medical disciplines."[88] They appear to have usurped the traditional GP role since many no longer have traditional hospital affiliation.

On the surface it seems hospitalists have been endowed by institutions to advance patient care and in the process assure maximum utilization of services and the highest procurement of hospital profits. They emerge to focus splendidly on the pursuit of profits by maximizing the economy of time and the utilization of facilities, perhaps less effectively when it comes to personalized services for the patient; in my case, at least on this occasion, that appeared secondary.

Interestingly, when the hospitalist summarized the NG tube experience in my official record, he noted that "the patient had failed" the insertion attempt five times; that was officially recorded as his professional appraisal of my NG episode. I had been through that unpleasant experience enough to recognize an attendant who was ill-prepared to perform adequately. The alleged failures in my

---

[88] Society of Hospital Medicine, "Definition of a Hospitalist and Hospital Medicine." accessed April 25, 2014, http://www.hospitalmedicine.org/ AM/Template.cfm?Section=Hospitalist_Definition&Template=/CM/ HTMLDisplay.cfm&ContentID=24835.

medical record are characteristic of the routine denial or obfuscation of unsuccessful medical performances. We now call it concealment, and most in and out of the profession now regard it as a serious problem. The physician must have recognized—but could not bring himself to candidly admit—the failure of his supporting staff with this procedure. It leaves me a bit apprehensive about other limitations and failures he or they would not admit. That cloaked behavior endangers all of us.

In *Complications,* Dr. Atul Gawande describes urging an inexperienced resident to attempt a new central line change in an emaciated elderly male patient where a slight error could puncture his lung and kill him. The defense—not at all convincing—is that that's the way medicine does it. "See one, do one, teach one, the saying goes, and it is only half in jest," he writes.[89] Lots of residents practice that abbreviated preparation, and a lot of patients suffer—and some die—because of that hasty pursuit of incompetence. One cannot easily miss the thinly disguised arrogance in this medical propaganda. Not too subtly implied is this message: "We are superbly competent, bordering on omnipotent. We master these difficult and risky procedures immediately." No, they don't, and the mortality stats attest to that.

As described in Gawande's book, the intern makes several failed attempts on the very frail and critically ill elderly patient. It is painful to read when you have been there as a patient. One cannot help but be highly critical of this. Transparency will shed light on this and help to reform this flawed system. I have been on the wounded end of bungled attempts by incompetent medical practitioners too often to be assured by their failing fakery.

---

[89]   Gawande, *Complications,* p. 33

For me as a patient, the attempt to insert the NG tube five different times back-to-back was an ordeal. Each failed attempt on the part of the inexperienced and incompetent attendant was very painful and resembled the experience and fear of suffocation. Again, get it right the first time. If you can't, seek out more training in preparation, please, before you are turned loose on suffering patients.

Dr. Ruggieri's cautionary take on the newly minted practitioner, the hospitalist, is illuminating:

> Despite the break in continuity of care, hospitalists are necessary and have become a standard of medical care today. They are one answer to the growing shortage of primary care physicians in this country. Yet with hospitalists the care by a long-standing family doctor is broken. Each day in the hospital, you see a different face, a different hospitalist who was given a report on your condition by the preceding hospitalist. As a patient, you get handed off. . . . With the handoffs comes the potential for breakdowns in communication. With breakdowns in communication comes the potential for medical errors.[90]

My Midnight Ride

Post-surgery recovery left me with chronic hiccups for several hours at a time.

The only temporary remedy was to lie flat of my back, perfectly still, and hold my breath as long as possible. After multiple attempts, I would shed them but only momentarily. They would return if I engaged in conversation of any duration. While in this state, a writing pad was my means of communicating with nurses and family.

---

[90]   Ruggieri, *Confessions*, p. 244.

I requested a medication for relief, Chlorpromazine, classified as an antipsychotic, which had been effective for quieting my hiccups on previous occasions. It was difficult to get a doctor to prescribe it. Most have little or no regard for this as a hiccup remedy. The standard response to my request was that there was no medicine for hiccups. They assigned me to a room normally utilized as an ICU until it was determined I had recuperated sufficiently and the hospital had a private room available for me. The ICU room assignment resulted from space limitations and was regarded as temporary. However, I did not relish being awakened and moved at midnight having been through a rough day in recovery.

Demolition Derby

I was awakened abruptly near midnight, after an especially long bout with hiccups, only to be informed that I was being transferred immediately—because they had need of the room I was in. I objected, but with little energy and even less influence, I was within minutes hoisted on a gurney and whisked swiftly down the corridor. Passing the darkened and vacant information station, we turned sharply into a hallway at a rapid and risky gait. I registered my displeasure to the young attendant recklessly motoring me about. As I commented on the late interruption, he became orally abusive.

After a couple of quick, jerky turns, the gurney crashed headlong into the exterior of the elevator, giving me a solid jolt, and my incorrigible attendant, a sharp nudge back to his senses. Immediately, he became excessively polite, a totally changed person. Any psychotherapist would have been impressed with the dazzling change potential of a crashing gurney at midnight. I concluded later that he might have worried that the episode had been captured on a monitoring camera. Transparency, remember, can be a helpful regulator even, or especially, in the medical community with its proficiently implemented code of concealment. Jolted from the elevator collision, but with little apparent damage done to me or the speeding gurney, I was deposited in a prearranged private area.

Bewildered Nurse

Arriving at my new location, I was foisted upon a kind, though sleepy, elderly woman, who described herself as a substitute nurse. She was alert enough to be troubled and disconcerted by the complex array of intravenous attachments accompanying me. She had no expertise for connecting me, nor did she know what to do, how to proceed, or whom to contact. Red alert!

This was just another of the many careless and risky maneuvers that could have spelled disaster for me under their care. I reached my wife by phone. After shepherding me through repeated surgeries, she was immediately aware of the danger and headed for the hospital as soon as she learned of my midnight ride. When she arrived, she buzzed the head nurse for assistance. Within the hour we had someone dispatched who was familiar enough with the medical and technical needs to restore my intravenous connections and avert a near catastrophe. Her arrival and intervention may have prevented my becoming another tragic, statistical medical error quietly ensconced within the cloak of concealment.

In reality, as increasing transparency will come to reveal, this was gross medical negligence. In my own case, these bizarre events occurred too frequently under the hospitalist's watch. His record with me, if indeed he was in charge, was neither comforting nor reassuring. If he was not in charge, who was? The profession should wrestle with that dilemma. So very frequently no one is in charge.

A final example of my experience with my first hospitalist occurred shortly thereafter. A nurse approached me early in the morning and said, "I hear you'll be leaving us today." Up to that point, nothing regarding my discharge had been shared with me. Given the fact that I was on total intravenous support, a properly graduated diet was an issue of concern. At noon that same day, I received a lunch tray fit for a hungry, active, healthy adult, piled with spaghetti and meatballs and other robust dietary items fit for one bulking up for a triathlon.

When the meal was served, the surgeon's assistant, a dietitian, and an ostomy specialist were present. All raised their voices in unrelenting and uniform protest: "He has to begin a liquid diet first," they said. The hospitalist was outnumbered and perhaps outranked but definitely outflanked. He rescinded his menu directive, and I was spared the potential consequences of his premature and unreasonable dietary order. And the rumor of my leaving turned out to be just that—a rumor.

Whatever priorities were driving the hospitalist's behavior, obviously my personal well-being did not rank near the top of the list. The hospital extended my stay a couple of days in order to adopt an incremental, responsibly progressive dietary measure to move me from a liquid to a solid menu.

Excellent Hospitalists

This particular doctor's performance was not representative of all hospitalists, given my limited experience. Two subsequent

Medical Madness

hospitalists attending me during my takedown surgery in the fall of 2011 were exceptional. They were both excellent, responsible and caring, and paid special attention to recommendations from a team of professionals assisting me. However, one of the three performing unfavorably in a life-and-death arena seems hardly praiseworthy when mistakes can kill.

Chapter Twenty-Six

Killing or Healing

Promise and Perils of Transparency

Speculation concerning who said or did what, without regard to whether or not it is fundamentally true, depletes our pursuit of honesty and integrity. Here we need an affirmation we can trust. We can be both precise and concise in communicating, not simply to be understood, but on a higher level, to achieve transparent clarity, so that we cannot be misunderstood. Now, we can begin the journey to trust.

Recent political discourse can be touted as an example: a surge of money has flooded the political process, requiring little or no accountability as to who contributed what. This further strains our troubled system. Wholesale corruption lurks just around the corner. Many feel the Supreme Court made a serious mistake with *Citizens United*, when they determined that a spigot of unlimited money was acceptable with virtually no accountability demanded. Money can buy access and power. What does that tell us about ourselves? What does that convey to the world about our country? Money means far more than it should. Profit cannot be an end in itself. How are we regarded compared to other nations on this score?

According to Fred Wertheimer, in an article entitled "Legalized Bribery" published in *Politico*:

Exactly four years ago, the U.S. Supreme Court changed the landscape of American politics—and in ways we have yet to understand fully. In its 5-to-4 decision in *Citizens United v. FEC*, the court struck down the longstanding ban on corporate expenditures in federal elections, a move that reversed its position on how corporate money enters the political system and created new avenues for corrupting our government.[91]

Each time I think the highest court in the land has pulled its last puzzling directive by flooding our elective process with unbelievable mounds of money, we get another shock.

"We live in the United States of America, Inc., where everything is for sale." stated Barry Levinson, Academy Award–winning director, screenwriter, and producer. He, in a tongue-in-cheek expression, suggested attaching notable business names to monuments and government buildings for a price. Then he said: "The Supreme Court may already be sold, but the naming rights are available."[92]

I am addressing this because the impact may be beyond comprehension for our democracy. It goes well beyond tagging the buildings; the goal is to be in command of the freedom of the people. Yes, you are your brother's keeper rather than your brother's brother. Money is speech, used cleverly, deceptively, to accomplish that carefully premeditated purpose—dominating ones' fellow citizens while masquerading as the constitutional guarantor of the freedom of speech. That the money/speech conundrum can shatter the eardrums of reason if they are prone to a bit of social madness. Power calculated in dominating decibels is purposeful. The Supreme Court appears to

---

[91] Fred Wertheimer, "Legalized Bribery: Four Years on, *Citizens United* Is Ruining Democracy. Here's How to Get It Back." *POLITICO*, January 14, 2014.

[92] Barry Levinson, "The United States of America, Incorporated," *Huffington Post*, April 8, 2014.

favor freedom via wealth more than equality. "All men are created equal" is much more difficult to hear when it is drowned out by the megaphones of dollar dominance. Inherited wealth may provide that road to royalty, coveted by our billionaire ideologues, which the Supreme Court seems determined to usher in.

Transparency International consists of more than one hundred chapters—locally established, independent organizations—called upon to fight corruption in respective countries. Transparency International releases an annual Corruption Perceptions Index (CPI) that ranks countries based on how corrupt their public sector is perceived to be.

Denmark, Finland, and New Zealand topped the rankings (the least corrupt, according to public perception). Almost 70 percent of ranked countries score less than 50 (out of 100), with Somalia, Afghanistan, and North Korea tied for last. The United States ranks nineteenth.

According to Britain's *Guardian* newspaper, in 2012 the corruption score for the United States moved up considerably:

> North Korea is still officially considered the world's most corrupt country, along with Somalia and Afghanistan. But why has the US gone up six places and the UK's score worsened? See how the annual corruption index has changed.
> . . . The US has had a larger rise though—up five places to number 19, in contrast to the UK's drop of one place to bottom at number 18. [93]

Ethical concerns about corruption loom large in America, as they should, and it is safe to say they always have. Note a very early

---

[93] Simon Rogers, "Corruption Index 2012 from Transparency International: Find Out How Countries Compare," Datablog (*Guardian* blog), December 5, 2012.

example from Alexis de Tocqueville, a French aristocrat visiting America in the 1830s. That trip resulted in his unrivaled classic *Democracy in America*. He made a strong but favorable contrast as he defined our young nation, paralleling it with his own country and the French aristocracy during that same period. According to Tocqueville:

> Regarding Corruption and Vices of Rulers and the Effect on Public Morality. Moreover, there is less reason to fear the sight of the immorality of the great than that of the immorality leading to greatness. In democracies private citizens see men rising from their ranks and attaining wealth and power in a few years; that spectacle excites their astonishment and their envy; they wonder how he who was their equal yesterday has today won the right to command them. . . . They therefore regard some of his vices as the main cause thereof, and often they are correct in this view. In this way there comes about an odious mingling of the conceptions of baseness and power, of unworthiness and success, and of profit and dishonor.[94]

We have, to our credit, elevated the ethics of human rights as a mantra and goal for America. We regard it as a symbol of acceptance for others and maintain it as a commendable humanitarian goal. We approve or disapprove of other nations vis-à-vis this stress test of basic values. They are scolded when they appear to fall outside our expected parameters of progress. Oversimplifying, it comes down to whether their citizens have been vested with the autonomy to know and the freedom to communicate and debate their countries' official positions and policies, as well as the performance of their leaders.

---

[94]   Alexis de Tocqueville, *Democracy in America*, ed. by J. P. Mayer, trans. by George Lawrence (New York: Harper and Row Inc., 1969 ed.), p. 220–21.

Preaching and Practicing

What is clear upon reflection is that we can do better to cultivate among ourselves a more highly informed citizenry entrusted with important facts essential for our country and the status of our vital institutions. The "average" person needs to be more assiduous and nurturing, and encouraged to cultivate the ability to think critically. Practically, looking past the impressionable headlines, we must parse propaganda and chameleonic camouflage and embrace our freedom of thought and expression. We must take hold of the right and privilege of a higher confidence in our participation. An important goal is knowing more about our country's intentions and actions. This is an inherent right, and at times it is followed by an obligation to criticize our own government, when deemed necessary. Transparency and accountability are essential for that procedure to unfold, and when that process is precluded, we have a right to be openly expressive. Concealment of unethical conduct should not be an option.

Trust is a conclusion derived from shared, verified experience. Trust will always be a consequential and substantial outcome empowering us and our basic institutions. We can't have effective policy implementation without it. A behavior is not validated by virtue of who commits it or who gets by with it. The notion of American exceptionalism, if not informed by this somber premise and calibrated by our reason, can distort our sense of justice and fairness, encouraging us to think, *It's OK only when we do it.* Justifying myself to myself puts prejudice over principle. Let's advance our collective criteria of short- and long-term consequences that support individual and collective well-being. Transparency will not be totally free of fault, but it does seem to strengthen more democratically minded societies, leaving fewer places to hide prejudice and bigotry.

To construct a cultural schema in which the enhancement of one's own group is central, and all others are calibrated with reference to it, limits the opportunity for inclusion and diversity. Locking into a belief in the superiority of one's own group, while harboring a veiled disdain for outsiders, fosters a presumption of inherited integrity. Assuming we are hallowed via heritage makes our culture the universal yardstick of values—unexamined and unjustified. Justification through inheritance is the opposite of achievement via wisdom. Not only is this riding the chariot of common sense, it has religious merit.

We do not dare to classify or compare ourselves with some who commend themselves. When they measure themselves by themselves and compare themselves with themselves, they are not wise.
—2 Corinthians 10:12 (New International Version)

The assumption of superiority creates an exclusive circular frame of reference as opposed to an inclusive frame of reference. Small gestures may serve to enhance awareness. The British driver navigates on the "wrong side" of the road. Why not just say it's "opposite ours"? Written Hebrew is read "backward." Why not just say "from right to left"? These are not mundane markers but cautionary symbols affording others the dignity they deserve.

Trust and the Vanishing Middle Class

The evaporation of institutional trust has been impacting the middle and lower classes for several decades. It is not a myth that equality of opportunity has become increasingly elusive. George Packer, a staff writer at the *New Yorker*, is the author, most recently, of *The Unwinding: An Inner History of the New America*. In a *New York Times* article, "Celebrating Inequality," he writes:[95]

> As mindless diversions from a sluggish economy and chronic malaise, the new aristocrats play a useful role. But their advent suggests that, after decades of widening income gaps, unequal distributions of opportunity and reward, and corroding public institutions, we have gone back to Gatsby's time—or something far more perverse. . . .
>
> One virtue of those hated things called bureaucracies is that they oblige everyone to follow a common set of rules, regardless of station or background; they are inherently equalizing. . . . Celebrities either buy institutions, or "disrupt" them.
>
> After all, if you are the institution, you don't need to play by its rules.

Mr. Packer goes on to lament the rapid vanishing of the once vital and sturdy middle class, which has been muscled out of its role as soldiers of production by technology, globalization, and corporations. Takeover artists—often utilizing private equity investors prepared to feast off the fruits of innovation—can make more money than ever by applying creative destruction and often reducing employment opportunities for the middle class. Independent companies are bought, sold and integrated without regard for employees' welfare. And given the ruthless yardstick of the quarterly economic judgment day, those on the short end of inequality have in fact been shorted. They may be needed far more than the flash-trading-mania addicts realize. The vanishing role of ethics and morality in our society renders it unthinkable that we might assist the middle class in their struggle because it is the right thing to do.

---

[95] George Packer, "Celebrating Inequality," *New York Times*, May 19, 2013.

Mining the Past

The recently deceased baseball great Sparky Anderson said regarding the past, "I've got my faults but living in the past isn't one of them. There's no future in it."

But I would argue that a brief yet worthwhile peek into the past helps nudge us forward. This is hardly a pleasant reverie; reversing medicine is seldom an exercise in pleasantries. At a basic level I do agree with Sparky's observation; the future will be now when it arrives, so technically, it is really impossible to live in the past. There is such laudable and deserving emphasis on the Founding Fathers and their gift of a free nation that we risk idolizing that period and distorting, reducing or elevating it to a mythology given the impossibility of recreating it. Understanding that is essential for making sense of our behavior.

Challenges were simpler then, more comfortable to the average mind, as memory buffers reality. Events, stories, and recollections became enshrined and utopian. These narratives recounted situations that were transformed into historic events, more potent and mythical with each retelling. They finally take on a metaphysical dimension with the Declaration of Independence and the Constitution even being dubbed "American Scripture."

Past Perfect or Future Perfect

Pick most any anniversary date, reach back a century or so, and see how medicine, for example, was practiced; you'll get a glimpse of what progress means. Respect the past but don't live in it. Progressive medicine is for the future, and historic contemplation must drive us forward.

We need to know all we can, lest our history, embellished by oral tradition, absent factual and substantive roots, mislead us. Factual reality back there, accurately perceived, determines the validity of what we make of it in the here and now, and how we plan for tomorrow on that perception. These formational events bring substance to our current beliefs. That history creates our present political and democratic reality. Transport today back to whenever, and our search for equivalence, puts the burden squarely on us. Is it truth we are after here, or persuasion?

No doubt those who really founded modern science were usually those whose love of truth exceeded their love of power.
—C. S. Lewis

We are all tattooed in our cradles with the beliefs of our tribe; the record may appear superficial, but it is indelible. You cannot educate a man wholly out of the superstitious fears which were implanted in his mind, no matter how utterly his reason may reject them.
—Oliver Wendell Holmes, Sr., poet, novelist, essayist, and physician (1R809–1894)

We must carefully unearth those segments of our history just as an archeologist would gently brush the clinging soil from their treasured and delicate relics. No rough stuff tolerated here. No jamming or forcing or ramming or pounding today into yesterday or vice versa; that's a fabrication—just a story, forced to fit. It is not then the truth we seek but a contorted and, by delusion, comfortable and fabricated ideology.

We are then creating a fiction where facts do not matter. Then our democracy matters less; that fiction will not function. That is a foundation of sand. There is no room here for fiction. Our world is full of it, and we are serious seekers, building a democratic nation.

We must go back since it is a given that our very Founding Fathers have become, to a degree, metaphysical symbols too. They are cited endlessly as we build our future on the foundation of their sacred past. Our reverence, however, must not obfuscate their human endeavors and humanity. They, as we, were into nation building. That includes our three streets—Main Street, Wall Street, and No Harm Street. If we do it well, we extend that great heritage; poorly done, we betray it.

Who were they? A small group of wealthy land owners of great stature, who were creating a country by breaking governing ties with Britain, their own country. Their goal: to live, govern, and build lives of liberty and wealth, independent of their own native land, which they had outgrown and rejected.

Our Founding Fathers comprised a patriarchal society, and that is alluded to almost exclusively. Many institutions in various parts of the world confront that patriarchal hangover, and it is a detriment. Founding mothers deserve equivalent esteem, which they too earned through their quiet but constant interpersonal influence, counsel, and guidance. Male domination was the cultural norm for countries during that era. Society had not yet evolved to grant our founding mothers their due, and this didn't occur until the twentieth century when women were finally empowered to vote. Men were forced to relinquish some formal authority and accept women as potential equals. Their hard-earned right to vote gave voice to their wisdom and acquiescence with their grudgingly reluctant male compatriots.

Modes of travel, as with communication, are an important means by which to compare and contrast our past and our present since our democracy is now an information society. Originally, intercontinental movement occurred primarily by way of sailing vessels, and overseas travel could take months. Land travel occurred by horse-drawn carriage. Time and distance limitations somewhat curtailed the travel experience and stand in stark contrast to our modern era. One could cover only about thirty miles per day with a fast horse.

Our current communication, which takes place at the speed of light, was unimaginable to our predecessors. The revolution ushered in by the computer and Internet, while still in its infancy, has the impact of a benevolent tsunami—creative destruction, innovation, and re-creation. Historically, it took some time for information, important or otherwise, to move from one group to another. The speed of discourse could surely determine who consulted whom about what, how frequently, and with what outcomes. What was deemed of major importance was defined in part by those restrictions. Local resolution was the only practical course of action. No wider audience could be consulted regarding most issues. Limitations, as we would regard them in looking back, created and facilitated their structures and systems.

Medical knowledge regarding the existence and importance of microorganisms such as bacteria and viruses was as yet essentially unknown. Advancement in such fields was fraught with ignorance and superstition. Today's routine hospital infections may well have carried divine symbolic meaning with all the rippling ramifications and judgments consistent with that era.

Women died in appalling numbers during childbirth because the medical community did not, could not, understand, embrace, and practice current standards of medical hygiene. Yet some doctors still have difficulty with the discipline of washing their hands! Do we really want to go back there?

Surgery absent anesthesia? The very thought can invoke nightmares complete with blood, guts, and gore. It was routine back then. Volumes could be resurrected about those times. I am just illustrating for the purpose of understanding and differentiating between then and now.

So if we wish to go back, with understanding, we need to call on our leaders, who aspire to build on that foundation and call to be followed in that direction, to explain clearly what they hope to accomplish as they summon, exhort, and direct us to journey into the past to assure a more sensible future. It is really about our future.

What do we hope to accomplish when we arrive at our destination back there by reversing the arrow of time? Symbols, usually resurrected in the heat of political discourse, are not helpful if they cloud our understanding of the truth.

Selective amnesia can mislead. Cherry-picking historical relics for comfort rather than truth can trap us. Warm and fuzzy portrayals of a utopian, idyllic life, so much more desirable way back when, run the risk of being a distortion.

Transparency and Democracy

> *The institution of royalty in any form is an*
> *insult to the human race.*
> —*Mark Twain, author and humorist (1835–1910)*

Each individual in a democracy has significance, virtually unimagined, evolving from the roots of royalty The elevation of individual participation embodies the practical, ordinary, and even mundane as relevant when it matters to a fellow human being. How essential for citizens who have a voice in their government to know everything possible about the affairs of state and their role and potential involvement in it. As such, our democracy will flourish.

Government Less Than Perfect

Applying transparency in hindsight, we might ask how would we have fared with some of the big stuff. A few briefly recounted epic examples are worth considering from the recent past, scrutinized in the light of transparency and viewed hypothetically via hindsight.

Precipitating the Vietnam conflict, with the Gulf of Tonkin incident was an explosive condition that played a decisive role in the escalation of that divisive war. The subsequent challenge of the Pentagon Papers raised genuine questions about the failure of our country to assess this in an objective and deliberate manner since so much seemed at stake. August 2 and 4, 1964, were cited as incident dates. Two encounters were reported and assumed sufficient for President Johnson to address the nation on August 4, putting the country on red alert. The accounts have been dissected repeatedly and appear to lack the stature of a casus belli (a Latin term referring to a justification for war). I am not attempting to determine the veracity of the diverse positions, pro or con. I am willing to place a premium on transparency to bring a degree of balance to such historic decisions. The result: nearly sixty thousand dead Americans and a crisis of confidence in our government's relationship with its citizens. It takes time and renewed dedication for healing to occur and to begin regaining what we lost. Many would regard the Vietnam conflict as a strong contender for the mistake of the twentieth century.

Iraq's reported cache of weapons of mass destruction was later dubbed a "mass deception." The distressing absence of the casus belli approaching that unfortunate war is also crucial. This miscalculation catapulted us into a disastrous conflict, resulting in over four thousand Americans dead and over a hundred thousand Iraqi citizens killed or displaced. These incidents suggest the possibility that disclosures, prior to military engagement, could have saved our country from precious lives lost, lies told, and more than a trillion dollars wasted, money which was so desperately needed here at home.

"Rafid Ahmed Alwan al-Janabi, an Iraqi defector code-named Curveball by our CIA, confirmed in an interview with the UK's *Guardian* newspaper that he had lied about the existence of a secret biological weapons program in Iraq to initiate regime change."[96] That counterfeit disclosure was used by our government to help confirm their quest for war against Iraq. That deception helped buttress the US case for invading Iraq the following month. In hindsight, we might recognize that we learned a lot—but at what cost? Transparency might have disclosed that our government appeared to be looking for a justification rather than truth. How else might one explain such gullibility demonstrated in embracing Janabi's phony testimony about the phantom weapons?

If citizens had been clued in that our nation had chosen, behind the scenes, to fabricate the image of weapons of mass destruction to remove a despotic leader, how would that have been received? Arguably, our leaders chose to take us to war on what were marginally believable but fallacious pretenses. Perhaps there would have been no Iraq War, four thousand beloved sons and daughters would still be

---

[96] Harriet Barovick, et. al., "Throwing a Curve Ball at the Iraq War," *Time* 117, no. 8, February 28, 2011.

alive, and thirty thousand seriously injured would not have suffered their tragic, life-altering fates. Our nation might have found a better way and would have been more respected internationally. Add to that the hundreds of billions of dollars that drastically increased the terrible deficit our Congress is trying now to repair by cutting what are regarded as essential services here in our own country, and you have a situation that demanded more thorough examination.

Before I leave the subject of Iraq, allow me to present one more witness who is regarded as impeccable in trustworthiness and credibility. Alan Greenspan, chairman of the Federal Reserve of the United States from 1987 to 2006, laments in his autobiography:

> I am saddened that it is politically inconvenient to acknowledge what everyone knows: the Iraq war is largely about oil. Thus projections of world supply and demand that do not note the highly precarious environment of the Middle East are the eight-hundred-pound gorilla that could bring world economic growth to a halt. I do not pretend to know how or whether the turmoil in the Middle East will be resolved.[97]

If, as Chairman Greenspan asserts, the Iraq War was really about oil, tens of thousands died on the false assumption that it was primarily about weapons of mass destruction in the hands of a brutal dictator. I believe transparency might have helped our beloved country avoid a tragedy of massive proportions in lives lost and a trillion dollars wasted.

---

[97] Alan Greenspan, *The Age of Turbulence: Adventures In A New World* (New York: Penguin Press, 2007), p. 463.

Transparency to Our Rescue

Introducing transparency into policy verification would raise the veracity bar for our leaders as they forge plans more acceptable to the American people. Structured transparency, while at times confrontational and painful, may help build a more vital nation where our leaders are accountable for their decisions and strategies. This would most certainly be a more democratic country. We often exhort other nations regarding their commitment to democracy. We should be reminded of our need to continue to grow as a nation. We are evolving. Our founders would be the last to regard what they started as a finished work of perfection. The maturity of truth and trust as ends, adopting transparency and accountability as means, are tough processes; but we can't have trust, an indefatigable virtue, or a growing humanizing democracy without it. The community of citizens will excel in their participation and contribute to the wisdom of our leaders as they are more involved in such decisive activities.

On the topic of misleading leaders, I must ask: Would disclosure, prior to raising serious questions about the verification of facts, have altered our military history? We may be hopeful, given the potency of these startling components, when we have actual input at a more grassroots level before we engage in a war that we can't justify or finish. Politically, the enormous cost—trillions of dollars—appears to be precluding entitlements for the poorest among us. I say this with confidence in the American people. We are intelligent, not ignorant. Grant us the premise and facts via transparency, and we will rise to the occasion. Could we have been more misled than our leaders on these vital, history-making decisions?

When so many lives are in the balance, whether it be under the auspices of government-directed military endeavors, medical services with an even higher fatality rate, or fairness in the financial markets, the fundamental principles of fairness and equality must prevail. We are still a fledgling democracy, and our subject encompasses life-and-death decisions in unbelievable dimensions as we strive to grow. Note: I am referencing both Democratic- and Republican-led administrations.

Life-and-death illustrations were chosen since our health care system is about life and death, with one hundred thousand dead each year as a result of preventable medical failures. I see an obligation, based on my experience as a patient, to share in the quest for positive systemic change. My factual account would have been less credible had not the powerful voices from within the medical community decided the time had come to sound the alarm. They have saturated the airways and print media with a deluge of sobering, heretofore unheard-of encounters offered with a spirit of transparency and determination. The system is indeed broken, and the time for change has arrived. Fortunately for patients, those within the profession have initiated it.

The Golden Rule

I put forth the Golden Rule as a great first principle to influence the direction of systemic change.

So whatever you wish that others would do to you, do
also to them, for this is the Law and the Prophets.
—Matthew 7:12 (English Standard Version)

My Definition of The Golden Rule

As I put this forth, please note, it is a behavioral proposal not based on race, religion, nationality, or cultural parallels. It is not governed by emotional dimensions such as love, hate, like, or dislike. It regulates the treatment of others based on behavioral reciprocity. It is an understandable, interactive baseline of behavior that assures that the outcome of encounters with others will be mutually supportive. What a difference from the tragic hostilities we see that result in frequent acts of violence and revenge. The Golden Rule cancels the need for such behavior. It is a beacon of communal fairness returned, ticking through the millennia, enabling humans in their struggle to overcome prejudices through mutually accommodating actions, choosing inclusion over exclusion as they relate to one another by welcoming human diversity.

Its contribution and potency can be harvested; this functional reality is obvious in evolving societies. Me or "me-ness" cannot cure cancer; we or "we-ness" can. To go fast, go alone; to go far, go together. But to go incredibly fast—to break the sound barrier—alone will not do; we must go together in that instance as well. See where this takes us together. It is a profound regard for the compelling power of togetherness, nationally and internationally, whether the destination is the moon, Mars, or the miracles of medicine directed against Alzheimer's, autism, cancer, Parkinson's, polio, malaria, and on down the list.

Transparency is effective in calling on the collective conscience of the community enlightened by innumerable interpersonal disclosures and reciprocities. It is very forceful in a democratic context, since all are to be treated equally with assurance that they are playing by the same rules. Transparency is a thinking person's process and will enlighten as disclosures and discussions unfold.

Transparency as Seeing Through—C.S. Lewis

The penetrating insight of C. S. Lewis, renowned British scholar, author, and educator, conveys the danger of surrendering our human autonomy in route to abbreviated attempts at understanding and enlightenment. Lewis closes his timeless, celebrated book *The Abolition of Man* with a tribute to the potency of transparency. I would like to focus on his choice as an erudite and validating concept. His endorsement of its comprehensive value in man's relationships whether in Main Street commerce, Wall Street markets, or No Harm Street health care adds to its universal appeal.

> You cannot go on "explaining away" forever: you will find that you have explained explanation itself away. You cannot go on "seeing through" things forever. The whole point of seeing through something is to see something through it. It is good that the window should be transparent, because the street or the garden beyond it is opaque. How if you saw through the garden too? It is no use trying to "see through" first principles. If you see through everything, then everything is transparent. But a wholly transparent world is an invisible world. To "see through" all things is the same as not to see.[98]

First principles encompass the innate, self-evident, multicultural, and virtually universal application of the Tao that Lewis addresses in some detail in the appendix of his book. I recommend it as a resource for those wishing to study this important philosophical concept in further detail.

---

[98] C. S. Lewis, *The Abolition of Man* (London: Geoffery Bles, 1956), p. 55.

For us, the first principles of Lewis and the spiritual practice of Taoism are applications basic to human relations. They encompass all our institutions, expressed succinctly, in life, liberty, and the pursuit of happiness—our fundamentals, our Golden Rule, our Tao. That is, if you will permit me, the foundation of the city on a hill. When we declare these to be "self-evident," we enshrine them with the "first principle" status that C. S. Lewis regards so highly.

Mixing of metaphors configures the precision of Lewis's thesis in that seeing through is visual, while understanding is cerebral. But comprehending and understanding are vital, as democratic citizens can hardly have too much insight. The real concern for Lewis appears to be nearer the cognitive than visual acuity. It is a point I alluded to generally in a *Time* magazine forum decades ago while discussing a related issue.[99]

> Surely citizens in a democratic society cannot be overeducated any more than participants in a vigorous athletic event can be too healthy. Now I'm mixing metaphors—but it is a very important point.
>
> Understanding with wisdom is not invisible in a limiting sense and one cannot have it in excess when coupled with compassion. We are strengthened as a nation when the index of citizen perception, insight, knowledge and understanding is at its peak—lifelong learning, the accumulation of wisdom, is essential in democracy. We are more likely to move with, rather than against, the arc of history, to be validated by the unfolding future.

So this is not the final word. It is the endeavor of this brilliant man, C. S. Lewis, to take us as far as he can. This deserves our most sincere analytical deliberation. His contributions are epic, and I am in awe of his persuasive powers, having read many of his books

---

[99]   George Huber, "Overeducated" (Forum). *Time* 107, no. 16 (1976): p. 6.

and recommended them to others. Lewis has been celebrated by followers, including one who said, "He has helped make my religion intellectually respectable."

What he has tried to do in his cerebral treatise on man is to invite us to challenge ourselves with the authenticity of who we are, and the difference between that and who or what we claim to be, while learning to live with the consequences of our discovery. The three streets I address here are primary arteries of our cultural and social structure and in dire need of maintenance. We have heard from many experts asserting the need for the systems to be overhauled, because as demonstrated, they are in effect broken.

I have in this brief narrative questioned our leaders and executives, regarding their efficacy on realistic grounds. In covering the terrain I must ask whether, assuming their integrity, they are pragmatists or ideologues. The former would assert that it is right if it works; according to the latter, it works because it is right. I think it's a bit of both. As a citizen in a democracy, I'm invited to think, and I also implore you to think.

Things are not always as they seem. Conclusions derived enthusiastically, on closer inspection, via thinking, may not measure up. The system may not enable or permit it. Validation by endeavor and examples hasn't worked elsewhere, or has it? Does the stated purpose through the planned strategy and process achieve the anticipated conclusions?

Taking on ourselves and our groups with the invitation, even the obligation, to think is a crowning achievement. We have challenged the systems on myriad fronts and invite you to think. Democracy is a work in progress, and thank goodness, we will not all think alike—there is more hope in diversity. I recall an old cartoon from an unknown source that depicts a youngster frowning as he returns from school and laments to his mother, "We learned to think today, and it hurt!"

Those of my readers who have championed classical novels may well be among the most adept at critical thinking. *Pride and Prejudice* from the gifted pen of Jane Austen comes to mind. One cannot escape the education her perceptive cast of characters offers us regarding the complexities of living in flawed systems and the impact that has on us.

James Franklin in his comprehensive scholarly treatise *The Science of Conjecture: Evidence and Probability Before Pascal*,[100] points to Austen as an educator par excellence.

> The notion of probability found in the evaluation of historical evidence pervades Jane Austen's novels on persuasion, sense, and prejudice. The crucial chapter 36 of *Pride and Prejudice*, in which Elizabeth Bennet is forced to make humiliating changes to her beliefs in response to the new evidence contained in Mr. Darcy's letter, is a tour de force of the careful reappraisal of a belief system that has been based on a large body of evidence. As Elizabeth "weighed every circumstance with what she meant to be impartiality—deliberated on the probability of each statement . . . reconsidering events, determining probabilities," she came to see that her previous opinions of Darcy's and Wickham's characters were based on vanity and were now insupportable. Austen goes through each piece of evidence carefully, explaining its relation to the whole.

Hasty conclusions invite dangers on many fronts. Things sounding too good to be true require closer inspection. Political promises can be, when examined, the very opposite of what they seem to convey.

---

100   James Franklin, *The Science of Conjecture: Evidence and Probability Before Pascal* (Baltimore: Johns Hopkins University Press, 2001), p. 370–71.

Is that democracy or plutocracy? Inclusion or exclusion? Rule by big money or freedom of the people to vote undeceived and without harassment? The politicians who have sold out to their keepers should be voted out. The general who decides he must destroy a city in order to save it needs to be overruled and retired.

Lewis, in this context, offered a humorous illustration depicting serious thinking derailed: A frugal Irishman got word of an incredible stove that would heat his house for half the cost. He was determined to buy two—that way he could warm his house for nothing.

Historic reflection can be both wise and seductive. It construes a mental gymnastic of cumulative experience and superimposes it on our hard-earned wisdom. We walk back to a time when our earlier "innocence," uncontaminated by the change of the convening years, renders an advantage that exists primarily in our imagination. Multiple and subtle forms of forgetting contribute to our problem-solving fantasy, thus clouding our reality. Perhaps that is why we relish the past so passionately. The future is far more challenging and opaque; we never know what tomorrow will bring or, more importantly, what we will bring to tomorrow. That is what this philosophical excavation is about. Remember the fallacy of the two stoves. We are at liberty to impose on the huge canvas of life a vast array of probabilities that would put a creative novel to shame. To forge a future from a past that could not have been comprehended by eighteenth-century men, a sobering reality that we cannot predict even a decade hence, may give us the humility to quell our unlimited certainty when embracing the past as our future. These are our opportunities, our freedoms, or the captivation of our discontent.

No Harm Street: Origins in Mythology

Those with a classical bent who wish to pursue the origins of "no harm" in Greek mythology may wish to use this legend as a beginning:

> In Greek mythology, the son of Apollo and Coronis was instructed in the arts of healing by the centaur Chiron. Asclepius married Epione, who begat Hygeia (health). So successful was Asclepius in the art of healing that Zeus was fearful that he would make mankind immortal, so he killed him with a thunderbolt. Apollo retaliated by attacking the Cyclopes who had forged the thunderbolt, and Zeus was eventually prevailed upon to admit Asclepius to the ranks of the gods. . . . The serpent and the dog were sacred to him, and his symbol of the serpent coiled about a staff still remains as the sign of medical practice.[101]

You may have heard the story of the young man on a beach after a brutal storm who becomes intensely occupied with sparing the lives of hundreds of starfish washed ashore. They clutter the sand as far as one can see. He keeps reaching for them gently and, with great care, throwing them back into the water. An older gentleman happens along with a bit of advice. "There are too many for you to make any difference," he counsels. The young man glances his way, and then reaches down without breaking his rhythm, picks up another, and hurls it into the water. He turns back to the older man momentarily and says, "It made a difference for that one."

The Golden Rule is like that. Look about you; there are plenty of storms and casualties as far as one can see, but living the rule—not just talking about it—will always make a difference for "that one," whether on Wall Street, Main Street, or No Harm Street.

---

[101] Emma Jeanette Levy Edelstein, *Asclepius: A Collection and Interpretation of the Testimonies* (New York: Arno Press, 1975).

Epilogue

The Science of Medicine in Our Future

Constructive Versus Destructive Power

I am proposing a different view of wielding power. This undertaking will require facilitating a behavioral norm that invites peace, trust, and harmony among nations and individuals. Our time is limited. Our destructive technologies have outpaced our interpersonal capacity. We must learn to live with each other in the world we have now created.

Virtue of Violence

America's prominence as the world's single superpower has been sustained in part by exercising our influence through intimidation. The empire image fits us well. That tradition is as old as recorded history. Ancient texts are saturated with them. Mythologies marched under multiple deities, and the most powerful gods were the victors, and their devotees, having sacrificed, amassed the spoils. No strategy was too brutal or devious. Winning was all that mattered—winning was survival. As an empire, we are their systemic heirs. Common attributes persist along with the antiquated dominating tendencies. Most with uncanny consistency, having adopted that profile, met with a comparable fate. Are we, too, destined to conquer, maintain, decline, and then collapse? Empires do not last. They are fundamentally flawed—predictably so. Check out our national DNA; a somber warning was given by a president, in a position to know, to warn us about "the military industrial complex."[102]

Current conditions here and abroad indicate time appears to be running out on our own empire. Intoxicated by our power, we seem insensitive to the danger as we plow ahead with repetitious abandon.

Medical Science and Military Science

Maybe there is a better way—a cure, if you will. A different approach to exercising power and influence may be far more durable, and with good reason. This is not medical versus military science but cooperative endeavors for the well-being of the nation and for the good of all our people.

I am advocating striking a balance between what I will call medical and military science. Heretofore, there has been little balance. It has been horribly lopsided. This is not for the good of the people; therefore it is not for the good of our nation. I am not advocating reckless abandon equivalent to parading nude in the Arctic while remaining ignorant and oblivious to the environment's impact on one's person.

Regarding other humans as our greatest danger could prove to be a fatal flaw but is certainly forgivable from an historical perspective. That is the way empires were built, lived, withered, and died. The empire emerges, as if from a cocoon, flourishes, struggles, declines, and finally meets its demise. The format is all too familiar: kill the inhabitants; take their land and possessions. Proximity and presumed power advantages are too crude for our more modern values. Having

---

[102] Dwight D. Eisenhower, "Military-Industrial Complex Speech," 1961.

become a bit more civilized and devious, we learned how to provoke conflicts as an excuse for aggressive behavior on our part. Would it be superfluous to say that times have changed and now we must change? We cannot control wars, even the ones we start. We should do everything within our power to prevent them. That does not fit the traditional formula for empires.

Wars Do Not Work

I'm sure that someday children in schools will study the history of the men who made war as you study an absurdity. They'll be shocked, just as today we're shocked with cannibalism.
—Golda Meir, Israeli Prime Minister (1898–1978)

Conflict resolution must not evoke the killing of dissenters. Dissimilarity between diverse cultures is normal. Sharing our divergent ideas could become one of the primary ingredients of foreign policy for the good of all. The stupidest and most dysfunctional strategy going forward would be to withdraw and isolate ourselves from those with whom we differ. We need one another. The fact that we disagree on a principle or premise should indicate that we really require collective and representative input to fully understand and resolve the differences with creative solutions. The assertion that killing others resolves conflict will one day be regarded as inconceivable. We are still in the process of moving away from our barbaric past. Let's do nothing to retard that positive movement.

Our optimal future, I believe, is the very antithesis of the traditional empire paradigm and can be carved from the life-saving harvest derived from an enhanced pursuit of medical science. It is the life science and should be job one. Military science, as currently practiced, is more of a death science. History should jolt us awake.

What a Difference Time Makes

We must not compete with tribal killers by mimicking their ruthlessness; that is not who we are. That is much more like who we were in the Middle Ages. Time and experience are the culprits here. We have accelerated and left them struggling in their tribal disarray. Our attempts to assist have been to build a more robust traditional empire. Now we are stuck in the past; we made a wrong turn in our attempt to bring freedom. We forgot that quality of life has to be a vital part of our existence. The difference between equality and inequality must be democratically addressed and internalized. Alarms are sounding. Inequality is surpassing equality and is out of cooperative balance; this represents an ever-present danger for us and the rest of the world. In attempting to impose democracy, we have inadvertently stirred sectarian strife, as groups sizzle in inequality. Having sown to the wind, we are reaping the whirlwind.

Artificial fears are not constructive. What we are suggesting here is that it is necessary to minimize attempts to influence the world by coercion, threats, and fear. As if our nuclear arsenal, along with our unmatched delivery systems, was not sufficient to cast an incomparable menacing specter, we are also unsurpassed in the conventional arms race as well. I will risk a generalization: If it is a lethal weapon, we make it and market it in abundance. This appears to be a dysfunctional imperial addiction. According to an article in the *New York Times*, the United States dominates sales of weapons: "The United States already dominates the international arms market, with nearly 80 percent of the sales, and the State Department denied a mere 1 percent of the arms export license requests from 2008 to 2010."[103]

Periodically, I search the tea leaves of systems projection and find I have been directional in my assessment of our national drift. Let's take a listen to those who should know. Recently, David Brooks, a *New York Times* op-ed correspondent, sounded a rather somber note characterizing our international prospects. After delving into his subject of concern with a group of Yale colleagues, he discovered some rather alarming scenarios coming from his esteemed compatriots. Charles Hill, a former State Department officer, was executive aide to former US secretary of state George P. Shultz prior to his time at Yale, and offered this insightful appraisal:

> The "category error' of our experts is to tell us that our system is doing just fine and proceeding on its eternal course toward ever-greater progress and global goodness. This is whistling past the graveyard.
>
> The lesson-category within grand strategic history is that when an established international system enters its phase of deterioration, many leaders nonetheless respond with insouciance, obliviousness, and self-congratulation. When the wolves of the world sense this, they, of course, will begin to make their moves. . . .
>
> This is what Putin is doing; this is what China has been moving toward doing in the maritime waters of Asia; this is what in the largest sense the upheavals of the Middle East are all about: i.e., who and what politico-ideological force will emerge as hegemon over the region in the new order to come. The old order, once known as "the American Century" has been situated within "the modern era," an era which appears to be stalling out after some 300-plus years. The replacement era will not be modern and will not be a nice one.[104]

---

103 Editorial, "Shortsighted Arms Deregulation," *New York Times*, October 18, 2013.
104 David Brooks, "Saving the System," *New York Times*, April 28, 2014.

I would be as pessimistic as Mr. Hill if I assumed that the only alternative available was the unwinding empire's demise; he is well informed on that score. We are a great democracy. Creative innovation is fundamental for us. I am suggesting a conceivable change that would end that downward spiral, which appears to perch us on the cusp of a singularity as our nation heads helplessly into the voracious black hole. Scholars of empire are very pessimistic concerning our prospects. This article was so recent and relevant I felt a need to share it with you. My optimism is that we can break out of that empire mold and wield a new kind of power for the good of all.

We do now have the ability to serve the world and our own citizens through an intense commitment to medical science—the life science, commensurate with a balanced military program. Our resources then would be better invested, morally, ethically, and pragmatically. Again, we must not match historic barbarism—we've been there and done that and are uncomfortable when reminded.

Andrew J. Bacevich, a professor of history and international relations at Boston University and a retired, US Army colonel, in his book *The Limits of Power: The End of American Exceptionalism*, regards our eagerness to solve the world's problems by exercising military power as short-sighted. We create a void of insecurity here at home and leave a chaos of unintended consequences in our wake for the nations exposed to that power. He writes:

> Here we come-face-to face with the essential dilemma with which the United States has unsuccessfully wrestled since the Soviets deprived us of a stabilizing adversary—a dilemma the events of 9/11 only served to intensify. The political elite that ought to bear the chief responsibility for crafting grand strategy instead

nurses fantasies of either achieving permanent global hegemony or remaking the world in America's image.[105]

The "self-evident" foundation of American democracy is antithetical to empire building. We can come to that conclusion, or continue to pursue this road of no return enriching a small cluster of greedy war mongers blinded by their momentary madness.

The funds assigned to wars of choice can be redirected to eradicate diseases that ravage mankind worldwide; they are the real killers. This challenge may even compete with Wall Street for attracting the most talented soldiers of fortune to meet this new altruistic and pragmatic adventure.

The profit issue enters here since we have exhausted our resources killing other people who differ from us. If we survive as a species, it will be in large part because we have come to understand the real enemies and strive to prevail over them. The foundation for polarization should not be in the ideological trivialities upon which we have misguidedly chosen to center our attention. Race, religion, customs, culture, geography, and so on must not present routine directives for hostilities. This is vital in our focus on the Golden Rule and the cooperation it engenders as an interpersonal guiding philosophy for our democratic systems. The destruction of those with whom we disagree leads down that perilous path to self-destruction.

Bacevich turns to a renowned theologian for guidance:

Niebuhr once wrote, "One of the most pathetic aspects of human history is that every civilization expresses itself most pretentiously, compounds its partial and universal values most convincingly, and

---

[105]   Andrew J. Bacevich, *The Limits of Power: The End of American Exceptionalism* (New York: Metropolitan Books, 2008), p. 165.

claims immortality for its finite existence at the very moment when the decay which leads to death has already begun.[106]

We recommend the extension of our influence for the benefit of all humankind, of the cooperative and compassionate services residing in the life-enhancing power of our unrivaled innovative medical science. This can become a unique way of exercising power. Presently, we have the rather unsavory reputation of spending more money on our destructive military science than the entire rest of the world combined. That is no compliment for a humanitarian nation boasting a commitment to life, liberty, and the pursuit of happiness. Should we be surprised that the reaction to our country by many nations is veiled mistrust or outright hostility?

The timing is optimal. We have ample reason to modify our approach, given the stressed state of our own country, the weariness of war, and the military chaos in the rest of the world, derived principally from attempting to resolve conflict by killing those who differ. The lessons of conflict resolution by force, always precarious at best, demonstrate that there are no winners. Want a lasting standard? Try offering life rather than death—a peaceful and life-giving solution!

A typical description of an acceptable national image (in terms of the way the world should view us) is redundant. How many times have we heard, "We want our allies to respect us and our enemies to fear us"? The result is a world divided and in a state of turbulence. With do deference, such a posture is a vast improvement over the all-too-familiar doctrine of preemption, which, if practiced around the world would incite war on every border.

---

[106] Bacevich, *Limits of Power*, p. 12.

That was the Golden Rule in reverse—do unto them (kill them) before they do unto you. It is a strategy born of hostility and suspicion bordering on paranoia. How paranoid we become depends on whom we have as leaders. The "existential threat," imaginary as often as real, is invited to dock in this harbor of absurdities. Permit me a recent horrific example.

The Taliban attempted to assassinate a teenage girl, Malala Yousafzai, because of the power of an idea. They failed, and though seriously wounded, she survived, even more determined. Her notion that women and girls should have a right to education became her cause célèbre. To brutal men, relying on ignorance and fear as a means of control, she became an existential threat. In their primitive and barbaric minds, she was the equivalent of a very dangerous weapon that would be the end of their culture as they understood it. They would become impotent; their power and purpose had no defense against an idea whose time had come.

Before we bask in righteous indignation—how like our own ancestors in the Middle Ages!—remember this: Their decision to kill has been endorsed again and again. It is time to change that with the power of a better idea. We are not suggesting merely turning the page, or even beginning a new chapter. Let's try a whole new book.

War as Perpetual Motion

I can anticipate the protests, but we are talking about offering the world a life science, a commitment to championing health and wellness. Conflict resolution via understanding, compassion, cooperation, and service will be more effective than all the horrendous wars we have experienced, and this may help lead the future by ushering in a saner world.

We don't need the foolish to drive us into a war that the sanest among us cannot end. It is easy to provoke "by accident," and no one can resolve everlasting war. A war unleashed is the nearest thing to destructive perpetual motion. That is the alternative.

The superb power of shared medical science borders on an ultimate advancement for our culture. It is the benign "shock and awe" in which we can unpretentiously take great satisfaction. The world will laud the science of life if we seriously commit to it and demonstrate its efficacy by applying its fruits, first on behalf of our own people. That is the essential expressive proof that it works and we are serious about providing an alternative to global hostilities.

In the past many potent medical advances were deemed too expensive for all citizens for the stated reason that it cost a billion dollars of research to create them. The idea that new procedures are affordable only for the rich will not suffice. What is a billion dollars to a country that can spend upward of several billion per week on unnecessary wars of choice? Reforming our priorities may be difficult, but it can be done. That is the essential balance between the medical and the military.

Exhibiting that model, we may then find a more eager and receptive world. As it is, the world equates our pursuits with the imperialists of past centuries, a group of which we had become a part. Now we can become number one in service to life as well.

The Real Threats

There is a fundamental need to focus on cultivating cooperation among Homo sapiens. Let's promote a unity of purpose. Examples abound with similar opportunities and provocations, usually surrounding the failure of men at the delicate art of conflict resolution. It may help to identify an alternative enemy against which hostile humans, who appear to need an enemy, can unite. They are with us now, everywhere, numbering in the billions—crawling over our skin, in our digestive systems, in our veins and lungs. Our cardinal threats stem from microorganisms that can by stealth ravage entire populations regardless of culture, race, religion, or ethnicity. They are more ruthless than terrorists; they unleash pandemics, taking out millions of human lives. We do not lack enemy targets!

Recent events in Madagascar were driven by the historic bacteria that destroyed a third of Europe in the Middle Ages. The rodent hosts were generous, carrying passenger fleas about, enabling them to lunch on human blood and thereby transmit the lethal scourge. Now it seems a form of a more devastating strand has developed that is passed pneumonically when a sufferer is in close proximity to others, and can kill within twenty-four hours. Man's inhumanity again opens the opportunity for the lethal microorganisms to gain the advantage. Note that as we have been distracted killing one another, the resurgent bubonic bacteria has experienced a heyday!

According to a 2013 story by the Associated Press, "Last year, Madagascar reported 60 deaths from bubonic plague. Poor hygiene and declining living standards as a result of a protracted political crisis since a coup in 2009 are cited as the primary causes of the spread of the disease." [107]

As civil wars now rage in many parts of the world, people continue to be susceptible in part as a result of their roiling hostilities toward one another, which have left them deprived and vulnerable. A recently reported epidemic of polio has resulted in the midst of the distractions of war. Hostility among humans has suffocated reason and sanity. The polio virus seized the opportunity to feast on destitute, emaciated, innocent children. Remedial strategies and existing vaccines were denied as brutality and ignorance reigned in the chaos of these senseless wars, which attempted conflict resolution again through the extermination of fellow humans. The microorganisms are celebrating such utter stupidity. They are the real enemies of mankind, a fact we have yet to learn. How long must we continue with this madness?

Our enthusiasm for funding research in life science with a sum commensurate to that currently supporting the death science would make hurried headlines around the world. Might we hear the bacteria and viruses responding in disbelief? They have no national, cultural, or religious affinity. Freedoms, rights, and laws are dreadfully irrelevant. In order to accomplish this we must change direction and stop being our own worst enemy.

Political Wars

Historically, we were plagued by religious wars. Our Founding Fathers protected us from that scourge with a brilliantly crafted Constitution. Our addiction to the very mindset and strategy of war

---

[107]   Lovasoa Rabary, "Bubonic Plague Claims 32 Lives in Madagascar," Associated Press, December 20, 2013.

has led us to adopt an absurd model of political warfare against each other here in our own country. The results are disastrous, often masquerading under individual rights of various stripes. The very life science we seek has too often become a causality of our own internal war strategies and mania. Dr. Francis Collins, the director of the National Institutes of Health, NIH, has lamented that his work has become a victim of these warring political factions. This heinous strategy destroys our country from within as it renders us all vulnerable to the real enemies—disease. Medical research has been sabotaged by political gridlock as described below.

> Because of the sequester and the fact that the N.I.H. budget has been losing ground to inflation for 10 years, "we will not be able to fund 640 research grants that were scored in the top 17 percent of the proposals we received," said Collins. "They would have been funded without the sequester, but now they won't. They include new ideas on cancer, diabetes, autism and heart disease – all the things that we as a country say are a high priority. I can't say which of those grants would have led to the next breakthrough, or which investigator would be a Nobel Prize winner 20 years from now.

> Of those 640 top research proposals, 150 were from scientists financed in a previous budget cycle who had returned to the N.I.H. to secure another three to five years of funding—because they thought they were really onto something and a peer review board agreed. "Now we are cutting them off," said Collins, "so you damage the previous investment as well as the future one."

None dare call this treasonous, aiding and abetting the real enemy. In 2014, the NIH was planning to offer new money to stimulate research proposals in a dozen areas, including how to speed up the use of stem cells to cure Parkinson's and other diseases, how to better manage pain in sickle-cell disease, and how to improve early diagnosis of autism. All were shelved because of the sequester, said

Collins: "Why ask people to submit applications we would just have to turn down?"[108]

Our Political System, Too

It should be evident to all who care about our country and their own lives and health that what we are now doing politically is sabotaging our own life-saving science. Have we become so bizarrely disillusioned that we cannot see where the potential death sentence is coming from? Shall we call it national suicide via politics?

It is not too late, however. We can still wake up as a nation with a mere case of dry mouth and constipation; but if we persist on this course, the symptoms will become too serious, and the patient will not survive. We are destroying our own nation!

Extraterrestrial Existential Threats

Moving from down here to out there, consider another source, a bit more esoteric—in fact, extraterrestrial; those roving space monsters orbiting us with the tug of gravitational attraction can appear with virtually no notice and lay waste to thousands of miles of our precious planet and kill millions of people. They bear no hostilities, but by their random routes, interacting with other planets, they loom menacingly, leaving us always at risk of an ultimate doomsday wipeout. Their obedience to the force of gravity can accidentally target and destroy us. We are great pretenders and procrastinators regarding the elusive unseen. They are so far out of sight, so far out of mind. Championing that protective cause is not about to get

---

[108] Thomas Friedman, "The Way We Were," New York Times, Sept. 24, 2013.

one elected for the next term—and therein lies the danger. It is sobering to realize that our survival as a species may finally come down to politics. The probability of collision, while remote, is very real. We need to awaken to the danger and enlist our best science and technology for cooperative planetary defense. Again, we are lulling ourselves into a cognitive slumber by putting all our resources into deadly encounters over human differences, which in a blink, astronomically, would be matters for comedic patter—but there may be no one left withwhom to joke or laugh. This is our home with all we know of sunshine and birdsong. I speak for all humankind, not merely a tribe or nation. As solar surveillance has sharpened, examples of collisions depicting potential devastation are reported frequently. Approached diplomatically it is another opportunity for international cooperation—if we can stop killing one another long enough to get serious about it.

Knowing the Enemy

In February 2013, [109] dramatic footage was posted of the Shoemaker-Levy 9 comet colliding with Earth in the Russian Urals.

The Chelyabinsk meteor was a near-Earth asteroid that entered Earth's atmosphere over Russia on February 15, 2013, at about 9:20 a.m. local time, as explained in a *New York Times* article by William J. Broad.

"Wouldn't it be silly if we got wiped out because we weren't looking?" said Edward Lu, a former NASA astronaut and Google executive who leads the detection effort. "This is a wake-up call from space. We've got to pay attention to what's out there."

---

[109] Feodor Potapov, "Meteorite Crash in Russia: Video of Meteor Explosion That Stirred Panic in Urals Region" (YouTube video).

NASA estimates that fewer than 10 percent of the big dangers have been discovered and other private groups are emerging, like Planetary Resources, which wants not only to identify asteroids near Earth but also to mine them.

Dr. Green of NASA said the agency was preparing to launch a mission in 2016 that will fly to an asteroid and, in 2023, return a sample to Earth for detailed analyses. The insights are expected to help scientists learn more about the makeup of the threats whizzing through the cosmic shooting gallery.

"If you're going to protect the planet, you have to know your enemy," he said. "You have to get up close and personal."[110]

Top Priorities First

As a nation, our infrastructure is rapidly deteriorating as a direct result of misplaced priorities. We have spent trillions on unnecessary wars to kill other people. Opportunities for the middle class are vanishing before our eyes. A comparable disillusionment appears, with more chaotic behavior, in many parts of the world. This self-inflicted jeopardy must awaken us to the necessity of exploring better ways to pursue both American and international accord. Once we are convinced through experience that we have a gift to share, hopefully the opportunity for cooperation and collaboration will follow from the four corners of our tattered globe, with the enthusiastic consent and participation of other people, once they are convinced we do not want to bring them kicking and screaming under the rule of our expanding empire. We can make it happen. Most agree we cannot continue as we have. There is a better way.

When our medical research commitment rivals our corresponding military research, and unnecessary wars of choice are recognized for

---

[110] William J Broad, "Vindication for Entrepreneurs Watching Sky: Yes, It Can Fall," *New York Times*, February 16, 2013.

their tragic consequences and abandoned, we can begin to delight those wishing to join the conquest over diseases. If not taken seriously and conquered, in due time they will conquer us. Winning and losing will take on new meaning. The world may be more receptive to sharing the benefits of this life-saving science. That is the new formula—and it is so like the spirit of the Golden Rule!

A New Mission

Our country has for too many years boasted of the fact that we spent more on military pursuits than all the other nations of the world combined. Is that really something to brag about? That is hardly complimentary—a symptom of paranoia perhaps. Moving away from a decades-long obsession being the world's most brutal and destructive weapons designer, manufacturer, and exporter of death will not be an easy change. It has become our albatross. We should find that the grand exportability of life through medical science will be a welcome change. It will be pursued with much less conflict of conscience—and with good reason.

New Heroes in War on Microorganisms

Where are our epidemiological superstars? Is it the NIH, the CDC, or one of the leading university laboratories? An understanding of the lethal potential of microorganisms seems so absent from our awareness that we permit such ignorance, lethargy, and absurdity in our political system to obfuscate this vital defense. This is health science, is it not? It could fall reasonably under the umbrella of homeland security. It is the fundamental purpose of government to protect its people rather than enrich its elected officials. We all are at risk. The time has come to ignore the rants of the greedy grubbers for wealth and power. The train of civilization can be derailed by the ignorance and irresponsibility that would permit us to abdicate elementary health science from our culture.

Capitulation to gerrymandering, gun lobbying, blackmailing by tax haters, extorting absurd oaths from our highest offices under threats of the euphemistic drowning of insipid governments in bathtubs—they do all this without being laughed out of reason's reach! Seriously, if our national leaders must stoop to oath signing, let's call on them to sign an oath to eradicate diseases; that they might do with dignity and respect, rather than what borders on this absurdity of political blackmail.

A curious bacterial observation was reported in the *Wall Street Journal*, which noted how researchers devised evasive maneuvers as a defense. The variety of strategies microorganisms use to approach their victims were noted; then researchers deciphered how bacteria communicate with each other, in order to develop programs that could disrupt their processes. Even bacteria need to communicate effectively to achieve their goal of producing an infection. Maybe this discovery of essential interdependency by the smallest of creatures in their treacherous mission, should remind us of our own need for positive collaboration on complex human endeavors to achieve our worthwhile goals as a nation.

According to author Shirley Wang, new approaches to bacteria are currently being investigated:

> An unusual strategy doesn't aim to kill bacteria at all, but rather to make them less harmful. Since bacteria only cause infections when their population has reached a certain threshold, called a quorum, researchers are looking for ways to disrupt the chemical signals the bugs use to communicate with each other. Another approach aims

to neutralize toxins or disrupt other signaling molecules that are necessary for bacteria to be infectious.

In another study depicted by Wang, a biochemistry professor described a potential method of dealing with such toxic organisms: "'We don't challenge them to a duel but basically confuse them into not causing infection,' says Gerry Wright, a professor of biochemistry and biomedical sciences at McMaster University in Hamilton, Ontario."[111]

A science whose goal is to bring fundamental health and security of life to Homo sapiens will be regarded as applied utopia. Elevating our community to this vision of serious reflection will mean that money, plans, commitments have to be prioritized and redirected. Here we must become serious thinkers. There is a lot of money (profit) in war, and a lot of money (profit) in medicine. I maintain that economies must not be hijacked to direct profit for support of killing other people. We make a serious error in judgment by regarding people as mankind's most formidable enemy. Listening on a regular basis to some of our leaders emeritus, the only plan they have for solving problems is threatening to kill all who would challenge the United States or its allies regardless of their geographic remoteness or the substance of disputations. I am suggesting the exploration of another way.

That portrayal is an insidious diversion, fueled largely by greed, to support the ancient and outmoded machinery of traditional war. Eliminate that profane profit from war, and most wars will fade away. Proscribe war against fellow humans and eliminate it when at all

---

[111] Shirley Wang, "Antibiotics of the Future: Scientists Hunt for New Antibiotics amid a Rise in Resistant Germs," *Wall Street Journal*, December 16, 2013.

possible. The killer diseases will rise as targets around which nations can unite, focusing attention on their eradication.

Moving from the negative, we may decide to become internationally cooperative in the pursuit of health and wellness, a process that is exciting to contemplate. Contrast that with the crazy world we have helped create. It is time to cease pretending we have had no role to play in its present state. It is time, too, for medicine to move beyond its mythical past and reinvent itself. It is time to harvest the cumulative benefits of the revolutionary, evolving medical science. Just in recent years, astounding advances in DNA, stem cells, the genome, and regenerative medicine, to cite a few milestones, have revealed the astonishing possibilities on the horizon.

We have relegated to charities that essential funding for vanquishing disease, seemingly a tragic underestimation of resources needed, but one that reflects the level of our value confusion. We should be glad to have what the good charities can provide for noble endeavors. Understand it is but a drop in the proverbial bucket when measured against the incredible need. A reasonable parallel could be to consider funding the military through charities. Diseases are just as formidable an enemy. It will take a while for us to come to that realization.

An Enemy's List: Real Bad Guys

It may soon be conceivable to develop an international public enemies list of the killer diseases that plague us today. Tomorrow's diseases also need to be anticipated and prepared for. We are way behind; they reinvent themselves with ease, camouflaging against our most potent medications.

Can we now join forces in their control and elimination? Enlisting the United Nation's WHO in the pursuit of health appears to be a worthy undertaking whose time has come. The politics of this could enlist the best minds in pursuit of international cooperation with a higher purpose. We will succeed only with significant political commitments from many nations, even if it has never been done before.

The Role of Government

Our subject cannot escape this thorny, politically loaded issue for the role of government. Stated simply: the role of government is to protect the people.

We have performed commendably in the traditional capacity of being the world's unequaled and most formidable military power. The rest of the world knows that. Complex issues surrounding such power have been addressed. One area in which we are currently deficient is supporting and expanding the role of medical science to meet the needs of our own citizens first and foremost. In addition we must assist the world by playing a leadership role, making up for deficiencies in areas we all admit are vital to our security and the world's security. A recent *New York Times* editorial described this succinctly with the alarming title "The Rise of Antibiotic Resistance."

The World Health Organization surveyed the growth of antibiotic-resistant germs around the world—the first such survey it has ever conducted—and came up with disturbing findings. In a report issued recently, the organization revealed that antimicrobial resistance in bacteria (the main focus of the study), fungi, viruses, and parasites is an increasingly serious threat in every part of the world—"a problem so serious that it threatens the achievements of modern medicine." The report went on, "A post-antibiotic era, in which common infections and minor injuries can kill, far from being an apocalyptic fantasy, is instead a very real possibility for the 21st century."[112]

Tribute to a Genius

I have been fascinated by the life of Albert Einstein, as have many others. Having read four biographies on him, I deeply value his social insights in addition to his incredible genius regarding our universe. We stand to benefit from both. It is the social dimension that we are calling on now.

I was awed to learn that, when Einstein became justifiably disenchanted with his life and career in Berlin, he spelled out briefly the qualities he felt important in a nation he would prefer—how consistent he was even then with our concept of democracy. "As long as I have any choice in the matter, I shall live only in a country where civil liberty, tolerance, and equality of all citizens before the law prevail." He defined his terms: *civil liberty* implies freedom to express one's political convictions in speech and in writing; *tolerance* implies respect for the convictions of others, whatever they may be.[113]

Few of us would venture to improve on his judgment.

Allow me another brief view of Einstein's philosophy, which came later in his life, after the world had been introduced to atomic warfare.

---

[112] Editorial, "Rise of Antibiotic Resistance," *New York Times*, May 10, 2014.
[113] Thomas Levenson, *Einstein in Berlin* (New York: Bantam Books, 2003), p. 418.

For the remaining ten years of his life, his passion for advocating a unified governing structure for the globe would rival that for finding a unified field theory that could govern all the forces of nature. Although distinct in most ways, both quests reflected his instincts for transcendent order. In addition, both displayed Einstein's willingness to be a nonconformist, to be serenely secure in challenging prevailing attitudes."[114]

Interactive globalization is a relatively new concept to the degree that it has influenced decisively the social, cultural, economic, and political dimensions of our world, necessitating interdependency and cooperation.

Scholars will debate whether the state of the world two thousand years ago or earlier experienced significant integration of societies, yet as Einstein envisioned it, this was new. It was essential because of the accelerated potential for nations to threaten the very existence of one another and the world. We are all in this together and must share out of mutual respect for the good of all humankind. Welcome to the nuclear age! Our standard of interpersonal recognition and acceptance is the Golden Rule. This assumes a values dimension that brings civility and harmony to mankind. The more interdependent we are, the more viable it becomes.

In 1908, Francis Macdonald Cornford (1874–1943) offered us an antidote to our frustration and discouragement: humor. "Every public action which is not customary," he wrote, "either is wrong, or, if it is

---

[114] Isaacson, *Einstein*, p. 488.

right, is a dangerous precedent. It follows that nothing should ever be done for the first time."[115]

Einstein has offered us a transcending premise: Suppressing national prejudices as necessary, resolving boundary infractions diplomatically and meeting international needs with a spirit of inclusion. His insight is irrefutable and so prevailing that we need to be consistently reminded lest our habitual, historic solutions prove to be overwhelming and ineffective in our atomic age. Everyone must care about everyone else's existential needs. Einstein knew better than most: the nuclear genie is out of the bottle, and our world will never be the same again.

We know his recommendation, though prescient, is not customary. We also know that everything we think, believe in, and practice was all once done for the first time. A touch of humor may help us over some of the rough terrain.

---

[115] F. N. Cornford, *Microcosmographia Academica Being a Guide for the Young Academic Politician* (Cambridge: University of Cambridge, 1908). *Microcosmographia Academica*, literally meaning "A Study of a Tiny Academic World" in Greek, is a short pamphlet on university politics written by Cornford that was published in 1908. It has acquired a small cult following as a pessimistic view of academic politics presented in a readable and lively style. However, the pamphlet is best known for its discussion of such things as "The Thin End of the Wedge" and "The Dangerous Precedent."

Acknowledgments

Medical complications following a routine procedure were so severe it resulted in a series of horrific corrective measures exposing me to months of accumulated hospital treatment.

That experience inspired me to write this book. The difference between my expectation of a patient's medical sanctuary and our vulnerability there should awaken all of us to that dangerous reality. The book portrays as vividly as and honestly as possible—how one is more likely to be killed in the hospital than anywhere else on the planet. It is an account of how one who was taught to trust was awakened behind enemy lines—it is about survival.

My wife provided help, beyond imagination, interceding on several occasions to keep me alive through five grueling complication ridden surgeries. When it appeared I may luckily survive, we shared the process of documenting my experience in the hospital(s).

My daughter and two sons were godsends of inspiration and hope for encouraging a writing task such as this. They understood my conviction was to be a lifeline for others whose expectations were as naive as mine and to all who have not been awakened to this danger.

My heartfelt thanks to the doctors and nurses [names are not permitted] who were so genuinely committed, regardless of the system, we will remember you forever.

Two celebrated author/surgeons Drs. Atul Gawande, *Complications,* and Marty Makary, *Unaccountable*, have declared the system dreadfully broken and recommend remedies. Both are great books, and if you have any doubt regarding the seriousness of the problem as I have described it, check them out.

Our initial editorial support was Ms. Wendy Thornton, a founding member of the Writers Alliance of Gainesville (WAG), a gifted editor and published author. She demonstrated endless patience and vital assistance on a regular basis. We are grateful for her talent, dedication, and commitment to assisting me with the book.

There would be no book without my publisher, AuthorHouse. Nathan Draluck was their voice guiding this novice who knew less about book publishing than cloud computing. His was a tone of simplicity, accuracy, and patience. The quality of my book is the proof of his commitment.

References and Resources

Barovick, Harriet, "Throwing a Curve Ball at the Iraq War," *Time*, February 28, 2011.

Bacevich, Andrew J. *The Limits of Power: The End of American Exceptionalism*. New York: Metropolitan Books, Henry Holt and Co., 2008.

Bloom, Allan. *The Closing of the American Mind,* New York: Touchstone, 1986),.

Bowley, Graham. "U.S. Markets Plunge, Then Stage a Rebound." *New York Times*, May 6, 2010. Accessed April 21, 2014. http://www.nytimes.com/2010/05/07/business/07markets.html.

Brill, Steven. "Bitter Pill: Why Medical Bills are Killing Us" (Special Report). *Time*, March 4, 2013. Accessed April 21, 2014. http://time.com/198/bitter-pill-why-medical-bills-are-killing-us/.

Broad, William J. "Vindication for Entrepreneurs Watching Sky: Yes, It Can Fall." *New York Times*, February 17, 2013. http://www.nytimes.com/2013/02/17/science/space/dismissed-as-doomsayers-advocates-for-meteor-detection-feel-vindicated.html?gwh=96ED9F0488478124F4AE4609F63ECBD5&gwt=pay

Brooks, David. "Saving the System." *New York Times*, April 28, 2014. http://www.nytimes.com/2014/04/29/opinion/when-wolves-attack.html?emc=edit_th_20140429&nl=todaysheadlines&nlid=32436386

Chen, Pauline. "Are Med School Grads Prepared to Practice Medicine?" *New York Times*, April 24, 2014. http://well.blogs.nytimes.com/2014/04/24/are-med-school-grads-prepared-to-practice-medicine/?emc=edit_hh_20140429&nl=health&nlid=32436386&ref=healthupdate

———— "The Impossible Workload for Doctors in Training, Fatigue and Consequences—Kill Patients." *New York Times*, April 18, 2013. http://well.blogs.nytimes.com/2013/04/18/doing-the-math-on-resident-work-hours/.

Cohen, Elizabeth. "25 Shocking Medical Mistakes," CNN, Aired June 9, 2012. http://transcripts.cnn.com/TRANSCRIPTS/1206/09/se.01.html.

Cornford, F. N. *Microcosmographia Academica Being a Guide for the Young Academic Politician*. University of Cambridge, *Published by Bowes & Bowes Publishers Ltd, Cambridge* 1908. http://www.cs.kent.ac.uk/people/staff/iau/cornford/cornford.html.

Crane, Kristine. "Rural Areas Drive Region's High Cancer Death Rates," *Gainesville Sun*, March 24, 2013.

Cresswell, Julie and Abelson, Reed. "A Giant Hospital Chain Is Blazing a Profit Trail." *New York Times*, August 15, 2012. http://www.nytimes.com/2012/08/15/business/hca-giant-hospital-chain-creates-a-windfall-for-private-equity.html.

Cromie, William J. "Doctor Fatigue Hurting Patients: Interns Feel Guilt, Lose Empathy." *Harvard University Gazette*, 2006. http://www.news.harvard.edu/gazette/2006/12.14/99-fatigue.html.

Dowd, Maureen. "The Boy Who Wanted to Fly." *New York Times*, July 14, 2012. http://www.nytimes.com/2012/07/15/opinion/sunday/dowd-the-boy-who-wanted-to-fly.html.

―――――. "Hold the Halo." *New York Times*, April 24, 2011. http://www.nytimes.com/2011/04/24/opinion/24dowd.html.

Edelstein, Emma Jeanette Levy. *Asclepius: a Collection and Interpretation of the Testimonies*. New York: Arno Press, 1975.

Editorial. "Coping With Infectious Disease." *New York Times*, February 21, 2014. http://www.nytimes.com/2014/02/22/opinion/coping-with-infectious-disease.html?action=click&contentCollection=Opinion&region=Footer&module=MoreInSection&pgtype=article.

―――――. "Hard Truths about the Bailout." *New York Times*, September 20, 2008. http://www.nytimes.com/2008/09/20/opinion/20sat1.html.

―――――. "The Rise of Antibiotic Resistance." *New York Times*. May 10, 2014. http://www.nytimes.com/2014/05/11/opinion/sunday/the-rise-of-antibiotic-resistance.html?emc=edit_th_20140511&nl=todaysheadlines&nlid=32436386.

―――――. "Shortsighted Arms Deregulation." *New York Times*, October 18, 213. http://www.nytimes.com/2013/10/19/opinion/shortsighted-arms-deregulation.html?_r=0.

Eisenhower, Dwight D. "Military-Industrial Complex Speech." 1961. http://coursesa.matrix.msu.edu/~hst306/documents/indust.html.

Erlanger, Steven. "Taking on Adam Smith (and Karl Marx)." *New York Times*, April 19, 2014. http://www.nytimes.com/2014/04/20/business/international/taking-on-adam-smith-and-karl-marx.html?src=me&module=Ribbon&version=context&region=Header&action=click&contentCollection=Most%20Emailed&pgtype=article.

Fox, Justin. *Myth of the Rational Market: A History of Risk, Reward, and Delusion on Wall Street*. New York: HarperCollins, 2009.

———. "What Would Adam Smith Say?" The Curious Capitalist. *Time*, March 25, 2010. http://content.time.com/time/magazine/article/0,9171,1975340,00.html.

Franklin, James. *The Science of Conjecture: Evidence and Probability Before Pascal*. Baltimore: Johns Hopkins University Press, 2001.

Freeland, Chrystia. "The Self-Destruction of the 1 Percent." *New York Times*, October 14, 2012. http://www.nytimes.com/2012/10/14/opinion/sunday/the-self-destruction-of-the-1-percent.html?pagewanted=all&_r=0.

Friedman, Tom L. "The Way We Were." *New York Times*, September 25, 2013. http://www.nytimes.com/2013/09/25/opinion/friedman-the-way-we-were.html?nl=todaysheadlines&emc=edit_th_20130925.

Gawande, Atul. *The Checklist Manifesto: How to Get Things Right*. New York: Picador, 2012.

———. *Complications: A Surgeon's Notes on an Imperfect Science*. New York: Picador, 2002.

Goldhill, David, "How American Health Care Killed My Father," *Atlantic*, September 2009.

Gordon, J. S. *An Empire of Wealth: The Epic History of American Economic Power*. New York: HarperCollins, 2004.

Graeber, Charles. *The Good Nurse: A True Story of Medicine, Madness, and Murder*. (New York: Twelve, 2013)

Greenberg, Herb. "Part 1: Controversy over Surgical Robotics Heats Up." *CNBC*, April 18, 2013. http://www.cnbc.com/id/100650872.

————. "Part 2: Patients Scarred after Robotic Surgery." *CNBC*, April 19, 2013. http://www.cnbc.com/id/100652694.

————. "Part 3: Counting the Problems of Robot-Assisted Surgery." *CNBC*, APRIL 19, 2013. http://www.cnbc.com/id/100653176

————. "Part 4: Marketing Is Key to Surgical Robot's Success." *CNBC*, April 19, 2013. http://www.cnbc.com/id/100652922.

Greenhouse, Steven. "Our Economic Pickle." *New York Times*, January 13, 2013.

Greenspan, Alan. *The Age of Turbulence: Adventures in A New World.* New York: Penguin Press, 2007.

Gupta, Sanjay "More Treatment, Less Mistakes," New York Times, July 14, 2012.

Hartcollis, Anemona. "With Money at Risk, Hospitals Push Staff to Wash Hands." *New York Times*, May 28, 2013. http://www.nytimes.com/2013/05/29/nyregion/hospitals-struggle-to-get-workers-to-wash-their-hands.html?nl=todaysheadlines&emc=edit_th_20130529.

Huber, George. "The Church Faces a Never-Again Opportunity and Obligation to Serve on the University Campus." *Christian Standard* 516 (August 18, 1962): 4–6.

————. "The Need for a Campus Ministry," *Christian Standard* 23 (January 11, 1964): 7–8.

————. "Overeducated" (Forum). *Time* 107, no. 16 (1976): 6.

————. "The Pursuit of Happiness." *Seminary Review* X, no. 2 (Winter 1964).

Isaacson, Walter. *Einstein: His Life and Universe.* New York: Simon and Schuster, 2007.

Judson, Bruce. "For Capitalism to Survive, Crime Must Not Pay." *Next New Deal* (blog). Roosevelt Institute. Apr 12, 2012. http://www.nextnewdeal.net/capitalism-survive-crime-must-not-pay

Kabat-Zinn, Jon. *Coming to Our Senses: Healing Ourselves and the World Through Mindfulness, Lying Down Meditations.* New York: Hyperion, 2005.

Khullar, Dhruv. "Medicine Is More Than Carrots and Sticks." *New York Times*, September 19, 2013. http://well.blogs.nytimes.com/2013/09/19/medicine-is-more-than-carrots-and-sticks/?nl=health&emc=edit_hh_20130924.

Klosterman, Chuck, "Should I Protect a Patient at the Expense of an Innocent Stranger?" The Ethicist. *New York Times*, May 10, 2013. http://www.nytimes.com/2013/05/12/magazine/should-i-protect-a-patient-at-the-expense-of-an-innocent-stranger.html?src=recpb.

Krugman, Paul. "School for Scoundrels." *New York Times*, August 6, 2009. http://www.nytimes.com/2009/08/09/books/review/Krugman-t.html?pagewanted=all.

Landro, Laura, "How Qualified Is Your Doctor? Doctors Face New Requirements to Keep Up-to-Date to Stay Certified," *Wall Street Journal*, January 20, 2014.

———. "Hospital Horrors: Meet 'Shrek,' a Doctor Who Insists on Surgery in Every Case—and Has a Surgical-Incision Infection Rate of 20%," *Wall Street Journal*, October 3, 2012.

———. "The Secret to Fighting Infections: Laura Landro Interviews Peter Pronovost" *Wall Street Journal*, Mar 30, 2011. http://online.wsj.com/article/SB1000142405274870436400457613196318589 3084. html?mod=wsj_share_twitter.

————. "Surgeons Make Thousands of Preventable Errors." *Wall Street Journal*, December 20, 2012. http://online.wsj.com/ news/articles/SB100014241278873244616045781896439933 571734?mg=reno64-wsj&url=http%3A%2F%2Fonline.wsj. com%2Farticle%2FSB1000142412788732446160457818 9643993571734.html.

Latourette, Kenneth Scott. *A History of Christianity*. New York: Harper and Brothers, 1953.

Levenson, Thomas. *Einstein in Berlin*. New York: Bantam Books, 2003.

Levinson, Barry. "The United States of America, Incorporated." *Huffington Post*, April 8, 2014. http://www.huffingtonpost. com/barry-levinson/the-united-states-of-america- inc_b_5110348.html.

Lewis, C. S. *The Abolition of Man*. London: Geoffery Bles, 1956.

Lowry, Rich. "Pilgrims Planted the Seeds of America's Abundance," *Real Clear Politics*, November 26, 2009.

Ludlow, Peter, "The Banality of Systemic Evil," Opinionator. *New York Times*, September 15, 2013.

Makary, Marty. "How to Stop Hospitals from Killing Us." *Wall Street Journal*, September 22, 2012.

————. *Unaccountable: What Hospitals Won't Tell You and How Transparency Can Revolutionize Health Care*.New York, Bloomsbury Press, 2012.

Mallaby, Sebastian. *More Money Than God: Hedge Funds and the Making of a New Elite*. New York: Penguin Press, 2010.

Meckler, Laura. "Beneath Budget Battle, a Health-Spending Juggernaut." *Wall Street Journal*, December 18, 2012. http://

online.wsj.com/article/SB10001424127887324677204578113138571167514067²2.html?mod=djemHL_t.

Morgan Jr. G. Edward. and. Mikhail, Maged S. *Clinical Anesthesiology* (New York: Appleton and Lange, 1996). See also: http://www.manuelsweb.com/blood_loss.htm and http://www.ncbi.nlm.nih.gov/pmc/articles/PMC2918661/

Morgenson, Gretchen. "From Outside or Inside, the Deck Looks Stacked." *New York Times*, April 26, 2014. http://www.nytimes.com/2014/04/27/business/from-outside-or-inside-the-deck-looks-stacked.html?emc=edit_th_20140427&nl=todaysheadlines&nlid=32436386&_r=0.

Naik, Gautam and Lalwani, Nikita. "India Manages to Free Itself of Polio: Against-Odds Achievement Remains Fragile but Brings Global Eradication Quest Tantalizingly Close." *Wall Street Journal*, January 12, 2014. http://online.wsj.com/news/articles/SB10001424052702303848104579312453860810752?mod=djemHL_t.

Nocera, Joe. "The Little Agency That Could." *New York Times*, November 15, 2013. http://www.nytimes.com/2013/11/16/opinion/the-little-agency-that-could.html?nl=todaysheadlines&emc=edit_th_20131116.

———. "Michael Lewis's Crusade." *New York Times*, April 4, 2014. http://www.nytimes.com/2014/04/05/opinion/nocera-michael-lewiss-crusade.html?emc=edit_th_20140405&nl=todaysheadlines&nlid=32436386&_r=0

Ofri, Danielle. "My Near Miss" (Op-Ed). *New York Times*, May 29, 2013.

Packer, George. "Celebrating Inequality." *New York Times*, May 19, 2013. http://www.nytimes.com/2013/05/20/

opinion/inequality-and-the-modern-culture-of-celebrity. html?gwh=AA4675741673AE85ECAA9348AD4FE073& gwt=pay.

Pickert, Kate, "The Art of Being Mindful," *Time*, February 3, Vol. 183, NO 4, 2014, p.43. Time & Life Building, Rockefeller Center, New York, New York. 100200-1393

Potapov, Fedor. "Meteorite Crash in Russia: Video of Meteor Explosion That Stirred Panic in Urals region" (YouTube video). http://www.youtube.com/watch?v=90Omh7_I8vI.

Phillips, Matt. "Goldman Sachs' Blankfein on Banking: 'Doing God's Work,'" *Wall Street Journal*, September 14, 2013. http://blogs.wsj.com/marketbeat/2009/11/09/ goldman-sachs-blankfein-on-banking-doing-gods-work/.

Plumridge, Hester. "Drug Makers Tiptoe Back into Antibiotic R&D: As Superbugs Spread, Regulators Begin to Remove Roadblocks for New Treatments." *Wall Street Journal*, January 23, 2014. http://online.wsj.com/news/articles/SB10 001424052702303465004579322601579895822.

Polk, Sam. "For the Love of Money." *New York Times*, January 19, 2014. http://www.nytimes.com/2014/01/19/opinion/ sunday/for-the-love-of-money.html?nl=todaysheadlines &emc=edit_th_20140119.

Popper, Eric. "Errors Mount at High-Speed Exchanges in New Year." *New York Times*, January 10, 2013. http://www.nytimes. com/2013/01/11/business/in-new-year-errors-mount-at-high-speed-exchanges.html?pagewanted=all.

Rabary, Lovasoa. "Bubonic Plague Claims 32 Lives in Madagascar," Associated Press, December 20, 2013.

Rabini, Roni Caryn. "Salesmen in the Surgical Suite." *New York Times*, March 26, 2013.

Reid, T. R. *The Healing of America: A Global Quest for Better, Cheaper, and Fairer Health Care.* New York: Penguin Press, 2009.

Rogers, Simon. "Corruption Index 2012 from Transparency International: Find Out How Countries Compare." *Datablog* (blog), December 5, 2012. http://www.theguardian.com/news/datablog/2012/dec/05/corruption-index-2012-transparency-international.

Rosenthal, Elisabeth. "Paying Till It Hurts—The High Earners: Dermatology Patients' Costs Skyrocket; Specialists' Incomes Soar." *New York Times*, January 18, 2014. http://www.nytimes.com/2014/01/19/health/patients-costs-skyrocket-specialists-incomes-soar.html?nl=todaysheadlines&emc=edit_th_20140119&_r=0.

Ruggieri, Paul A. *Confessions of a Surgeon* New York,. Berkley Publishing Group, 2012.

Sack, Kevin. "Doctors Start to Say 'I'm Sorry' Long Before 'See You in Court.'" *New York Times*, May 18, 2008. http://www.nytimes.com/2008/05/18/us/18apology.html?pagewanted=print.

Sagan, Carl, (1997) Pale Blue Dot: A Vision of the Human Future in Space, retrieved from: http://www.goodreads.com/work/quotes/1816628-pale-blue-dot-a-vision-of-the-human-future-in-space

Society of Hospital Medicine. "Definition of a Hospitalist and Hospital Medicine." Accessed April 25, 2014. http://www.hospitalmedicine.org/AM/Template.

cfm?Section=Hospitalist_Definition&Template=/CM/ HTMLDisplay.cfm&ContentID=24835.

Tanner, Lindsey. "Robot Hot among Surgeons but FDA Taking Fresh Look, New York,." April 13, 2013. http://bigstory.ap.org/ article/robot-hot-among-surgeons-fda-taking-new-look.

Tocqueville, Alexis. *Democracy in America*. Edited by J. P. Mayer. Translated by George Lawrence. New York: Harper and Row, 1969.

Von Drehle, David. "The Robotic Economy" *Time*, September 9, 2013.

Walker, Joseph. "Intuitive Surgical Warns of Problem with Robot Tool: Instruments Used in Robots Can Momentarily Stall During Procedures, FDA Advises." *Wall Street Journal*, December 4, 2013. http://online.wsj.com/news/article_email/ SB10001424052702304451904579238182142888184- lMyQjAxMTAzMDAwNTEwNDUyWj.

Wang, Shirley S., "New Rx for Young Doctors: Shorter Work Day." *Wall Street Journal*, June 24, 2010. http://online.wsj.com/ article/SB1000142405274870390000457532513051102894 68.html.

———. "Scientists Hunt for New Antibiotics amid a Rise in Resistant Germs." *Wall Street Journal*, December 16, 2013 http://online.wsj.com/news/articles/ SB10001424052702304173704579262551354298622? mod=djemHL_t.

Weaver, Christopher. "Treatment Woes Can Bolster Profit." *Wall Street Journal*, April 17, 2013. http://online.wsj.com/article/ SB10001424127887324345804578426693303833964. html?mod=djemHL_t.

Weber, Max. *The Protestant Ethic and the Spirit of Capitalism.* (1904) New York: Routledge, Taylor and Francis Group, 2005. http://www.d.umn.edu/cla/faculty/jhamlin/1095/ The%20Protestant%20Ethic%20and%20the%20Spirit%20 of%20Capitalism.pdf.

Wertheimer, Fred. "Legalized Bribery: Four Years on, *Citizens United* Is Ruining Democracy. Here's How to Get it Back." *POLITICO,* January 14, 2014. http://www.democracy21. org/money-in-politics/press-releases-money-in-politics/fred-wertheimer-article-for-politico-magazine-legalized-bribery/.

Wilkinson, Richard and Pickett, Kate. *The Spirit Level: Why Greater Equality Makes Societies Stronger.* New York: Bloomsbury Press, 2009.

Winter, Roberta E., "Review of David Goldhill, *Catastrophic Care: How American Health Care Killed My Father—and How We Can Fix It,* (Vintage Press, 2013)," *New York Journal of Books.*

Young, Rick, producer. "Hunting the Nightmare Bacteria," *Frontline.* PBS, October 22, 2013.

Inclusive Retrospect and Further Reading

Medical Ethics

Gawande, Atul. *The Checklist Manifesto: How to Get Things Right.* New York: Picador, 2012.

Makary, Marty. *Unaccountable: What Hospitals Won't Tell You and How Transparency Can Revolutionize Health Care.* New York, Bloomsbury Press, 2012.

Reid, T. R. *The Healing of America: A Global Quest for Better, Cheaper, and Fairer Health Care.* New York: Penguin Press, 2009.

Inclusive Ethics

Constitution of The United States of America

Lewis, C. S. *The Abolition of Man.* London: Geoffery Bles, 1956.

Tocqueville, Alexis. *Democracy in America.* Edited by J. P. Mayer. Translated by George Lawrence. New York: Harper and Row, 1969.

Franklin, James. *The Science of Conjecture: Evidence and Probability Before Pascal.* Baltimore: Johns Hopkins University Press, 2001.

Financial Innovation

Lewis, Michael, Flash Boys: A Wall Street Revolt, New York, W.W. Norton & Co., 2014

Mallaby, Sebastian. *More Money Than God: Hedge Funds and the Making of a New Elite.* New York: Penguin Press, 2010.

Bacterial and Viral Infections

Superbugs

http://www.medicinenet.com/script/main/art.asp?articlekey=61933

Polio Vaccine

"Salk Produces Polio Vaccine 1952." *A Science Odyssey: People and Discoveries.* PBS. http://www.pbs.org/wgbh/aso/databank/entries/dm52sa.html

Transparency International, the Global Coalition Against Corruption

http://www.transparency.org/

Public Safety

Trucker Regulations

http://www.fmcsa.dot.gov/rules-regulations/truck/driver/truck-
   driver.htm

http://www.fmcsa.dot.gov/